MANIFESTING WITH VIBRATIONS

Find Out How to Raise Your Vibrations, Achieve Your Goals, Become More Self-Aware, Attract More Wealth, and Become More in Touch With the Universe in Only 30 days (2022)

Audrey Johnston

Table of Contents

Introduction

We are all a part of the universe. Some contend that God is the energy that permeates everything and that God is everything. If this is the case, then God is a part of every one of us, and we have more power than we ever imagined. It is undoubtedly divine to have the ability to manifest and turn nebulous inspirations into concrete things. You will learn about the true nature of yourself, this world, and the Universe in and around you after you take off your blinders and limiting beliefs.

At its most basic level, energy makes up the universe.

The matter is created from this energy. The several types of particles that make up matter are then converted into the elements. One electron and one proton, two distinct particles, make up hydrogen, which can be found to contain both of them. Helium would result from the addition of another particle to an existing hydrogen atom. So, one element comes after another. But energy remains the same as the initial position.

This was discovered by Einstein when he arrived at the equation e=mc2.

You frequently observe it and have seen it everywhere. You already know that this implies that mass and energy are equivalent. It is more than that, though. In certain states, matter and energy are the same things. It's similar to how water in different states—such as steam and ice—looks the same.

Ice appears to be a tangible substance since you can hold it, study it with your senses, and even count it. On the other hand, steam cannot be seen, touched, or measured with only your senses in the absence of any apparatus. Let's assume for this discussion that this water steam is intangible.

There is a similarity between energy and matter. Energy is not palpable while the matter is (again, in the absence of special equipment). You have the same body. It consists of both tissue and soul. The soul is not tangible, whereas tissue is.

There are tangible and intangible things in this world. The tangible are the components you can see, whereas the intangible are the components you cannot see directly but can infer their presence by the behavior of the other components or matter around them.

What does meditation have to do with any of this?

Silence is intangible, but the sound is tangible. So if we needed a neat little package, here it is: the intangible column is made up of energy, steam, and the soul, whereas the tangible column is made up of matter, water, and the body's tissue.

Because you can detect sounds with one of your senses, sounds are tangible. Because emotions are essentially chemical reactions in your body that produce a specific amount of detection, they are also physically detectable. However, silence is imperceptible to all of your bodily senses and is only audible through exclusion. Silence is therefore seen as an intangible.

Since they are ethereal, energy, the soul, and silence are all in the same column. We believe that the soul is a component of the universal energy that resides within us.

Therefore, you must use silence to understand the soul and, by extension, the Universe. But it's much simpler than it sounds to do that. Simply ceasing to speak or to listen is insufficient. It takes a different approach to invoke this kind of silence, and that approach is meditation.

The silence of the soul is obscured by the mind's diversions, which are in constant conflict with the body. You must mute the confusion in your thoughts to achieve that silence. This is the main reason why most people think that the goal of meditation is to quiet the mind. Before being able to enjoy meditation, the mind must be stilled.

The secret of manifestation lies in this. You must be mentally clear. Your capacity to vibrate your wants increases dramatically after you accomplish that. Your power to attract is more potent, and you have mastered the art of attracting opportunity rather than a distraction.

The way you conduct your life forms the foundation for your ability to create. As long as we live a life with positive vibrations, it is a gift that each of us has and not a recipe for making desires come true.

Resistance is characterized by hard labor and effort because you are conquering, giving up, or striving against something, and this does not feel pleasant. You should enjoy living! All you have to do is shift your perspective from one of resistance to one of allowing you to fulfill all your goals without effort, sacrifice, or difficulty. Go with the flow of happiness and well-being and allow it to lead you to where you want to go. Allow wonderful things to come to you freely and effortlessly.

Like any talent, shifting your thinking can be difficult at first, but the more you practice, the easier it gets until it eventually becomes second nature to you and operates automatically. You will start to think and feel more and more in terms of wealth and prosperity as you rewrite the neural pathways in your brain, and the notions of lack and scarcity will start to fade.

People frequently inquire as to how they can shift their perspective and begin thinking and feeling abundant when they are stuck in a job, despite their meager pay, are in debt, and struggle to make ends meet each month. They only need to look at their bank account to see how "non-abundant" it appears.

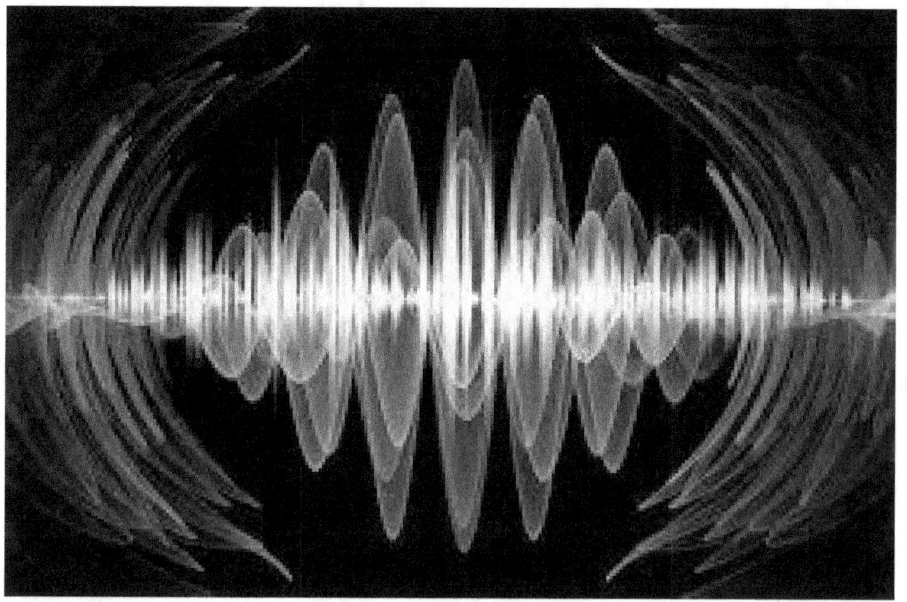

How do vibrations work?

We all emit vibrations, often known as "vibes," in everyday speech. When you first meet someone, you could feel good about them. What, though, are these vibrations exactly? Being energy, they. The energy at the subatomic level makes up everything in the cosmos. Our ideas and the forms of energy we possess inside of ourselves determine the types of energy we output.

We typically don't notice or focus much on this energy. But this energy is not simply a life-giving power; it also follows us through our lives. While other emotions can instill desired vibrations and thought patterns, some emotions can cause us to act in ways that we don't want to. If you click with someone, there's a good possibility you share their worldview, way of thinking, and self-perception.

How to Recognize the Contrast

The majority of us are certain about what we don't want but aren't sure what we do want. The two are separated by a different distance. It is essential to be clear about what we desire to direct our efforts and visions toward attracting it. How do we start the procedure?

Start observing the kinds of thoughts and actions that make you feel good or bad. Then, while you consider these various situations, take note of the discrepancy in your feelings and state of health.

Clarifying what you do and do not want in life requires this kind of awareness of your ideas.

Fear and Love

All feelings are ultimately reducible to either love or fear. Joy, happiness, contentment, pleasure, appreciation, and hope are examples of love feelings that provide an open, relaxed sensation in the body. Anger, wrath, jealousy, fear, sadness, and guilt are examples of fear-based emotions that cause physical tightness, pain, and closure. It will be simpler to invest in these concepts and experiences the more conscious you become of the thoughts and deeds that produce love.

Science has since disproved the ancient wisdom of the philosophers who held that nothing stopped and everything moved. All particles, large and microscopic, spin and move as a result of which they vibrate. Life itself is a tremendous vibration whose frequency varies depending on the type of matter it is.

According to the LOA, since everything vibrates at a certain frequency, objects with comparable frequencies are drawn to one another, much as in the phrase "like attracts like." When you are happy, more happiness comes into your life, and when you are sad, more unpleasant things come into your life. A vibration's resonance is its capacity to draw in other energies of a like frequency.

Instead of judging your energy, the cosmos amplifies what you vibrate or emit. It is similar to placing a restaurant order. Look at the status of your physical life to comprehend what you are requesting. ties, finances, and vacations? By continually deciding on different feelings and thoughts, you can always alter your order.

You can access a desire's vibration by considering its energetics.

Once you get used to experiencing that frequency, you start to resonate with it. What do you imagine the sensations of love and a million bucks to be like?

Spend some time each day honing your ability to visualize that experience. Always keep in mind that while thought and imagery produce the sensation, the emotion itself generates the vibration or energy. To tune into it, continually practice that, access the emotion, and take on that vibration.

like selecting a radio station.

There are frequencies everywhere. The million-dollar station, the station for love, the station for a better job, and the station for vacation. You must regularly practice tuning into the vibrations that are always present. gaining awareness of the feeling and associating your mind with the desired energy. When the meal is prepared, your order will resonate with you and be presented to you since the idea is the order and the cooking is the practice of the vibration.

The biggest misconception about the LOA is that people think it should work immediately if it's true. Ideas must first be chosen, then they need to be tended to and maintained so they can grow (imagine their regular fulfillment). The idea will come to fruition when it is ready to do so, much like a fetus.

Everything in the cosmos is interconnected since everything is made of energy. Everything—including the clouds, the water that makes up the oceans, the animals, the trees, me, you—came from one source and will eventually return to it. Energy also includes thoughts and feelings. Everything and everyone on this earth will be influenced by the thoughts and feelings you have. If this is the case, then since our minds have control over matter, we can build our realities.

This fundamental reality is supported by data from quantum physics. It is an enormous idea with enormous ramifications. If you try to comprehend it all, you'll get a headache. The majority of people don't even consider it. If you can incorporate the spiritual element into it, it does explain our fundamental existence.

This knowledge is useful since it serves as the starting point for understanding who we are and how the world works. This can help us see the wider perspective of life.

Finding a method to explain everything while not completely blowing your head and still making this knowledge helpful so you can profit from it is difficult.

You'll hear words like resonate and vibrations a lot as you try to make sense of it all. Simply said, this is a simpler explanation of everything. It explains how our senses translate everything around us into vibrations and how they do so. This is described in terms of "an invisible moving force that can affect our physical universe" by quantum physics.

It explains how we delude ourselves into believing that our senses can only perceive a limited set of things in the outside world. The law of attraction and your development must be connected once you realize that everything is energy.

Everything is energy, but our five senses are not entirely capable of understanding this. You can see it as an illusion once you completely comprehend that everything is energy.

Despite what our senses are trying to tell us, this is the case. There is nothing but energy, sometimes referred to as source energy, and it has a wide range of fluctuating forms and frequencies. The way energy interacts with one another makes the biggest difference.

You will never observe energy's constant interactions with everything. It's possible that you can feel this energy. Everyone is accustomed to hearing the phrase "energy in motion" whether referring to our feelings or physical energy.

The ability to manage our thoughts is a beautiful trait that only humans possess.

Everybody has the power to use their free will to decide where and how to focus their energy. When compared to the amount of energy we expend on unconscious thoughts, this percentage is quite modest.

This energy will search for a vibration that matches the one that our thoughts produce, which is an incredibly precise vibration. You won't even be conscious of doing it. This sounds like a tuning fork pinging. If it is close enough, it can induce an object with the same frequency to vibrate, and if so, it will be in vibrational harmony.

All energy in the universe vibrates, and every object has its specific vibration. According to the fundamental law of attraction, energy will gravitate toward other energies with which it resonates.

Everything in the universe, including its physical and nonphysical components, is just intelligent, vibrating energy.

Never does anything stop. Whether anything is visible to us or not, the key distinction between them is how quickly they vibrate.

Have you ever observed how events frequently occur in waves? A flood of emotion overtakes your body and thoughts as you sit at home contemplating something. A wave of heat smacks you in the face when you open the oven door. Thunder can be heard as a sound wave during a thunderstorm. On a windy day, you can feel the wave of air blowing your hair if you're outside. While working in the garden outside, you can feel the sun's rays interacting with your skin. The surf waves wash over your feet as you stroll along the sand. Waves will be created by all types of energy. This energy only changes forms; it cannot ever be created or destroyed.

Even thoughts have energy. The most potent electromagnetic device ever made is the human brain. You don't need to be a physicist to comprehend this, but once you start to grasp the idea that everything is energy, you'll see that you can translate it into terms you can apply to your own life.

Humans have free will and consciousness, thus there are many more levels to consider since we can form our views depending on what we were taught as children and on our life experiences.

This is our power, but it can be difficult because we oftentimes aren't even conscious of the limiting beliefs that hinder the flow of energy within us. Our belief systems, which are also made of energy, are what stand in the way of our attempts to draw things to us.

Because our belief system is only as strong as the energy we put into it, it cannot be altered. When you finally accept that your beliefs are false, such as when you say, "I will never find a job." You could employ treatment, such as EFT, to get rid of specific issues, such as "I will never be able to get out of debt," so that you can be open to new realities and opportunities.

You'll likely encounter some points of resistance that are neither right nor wrong. It only showed up as a result of your beliefs or current point of view. If you do locate them, think of it as a gift. Be aware of it and thankful that you had the chance to transform it into something you enjoyed.

Everyone vibrates with a particular type of energy, and we will draw that energy into our lives. Although we may believe that we are concentrating on the things we want, deep down we are vibrating, believing, and concentrating on the things we don't have. You will be able to take new behaviors and broaden the mind, which will then produce new results if you can get rid of your low vibrations and subconscious blockages.

Consider all the things you have in your life, including your partner, kids, house, financial account, and overall health.

All of these are items you have produced in your life. Now attempt to recall the main ideas and beliefs, and check if they still hold. If you're being absolutely honest, you should see a connection between how you imagined your life to be and what you believed was either achievable or what you believed you deserved and could do. You might observe that these limitations are reflected in your life.

You might feel more confident about your impending transition now that you know everything is energy and that you are nothing but energy. Give it some time if you're not sure you understand it yet.

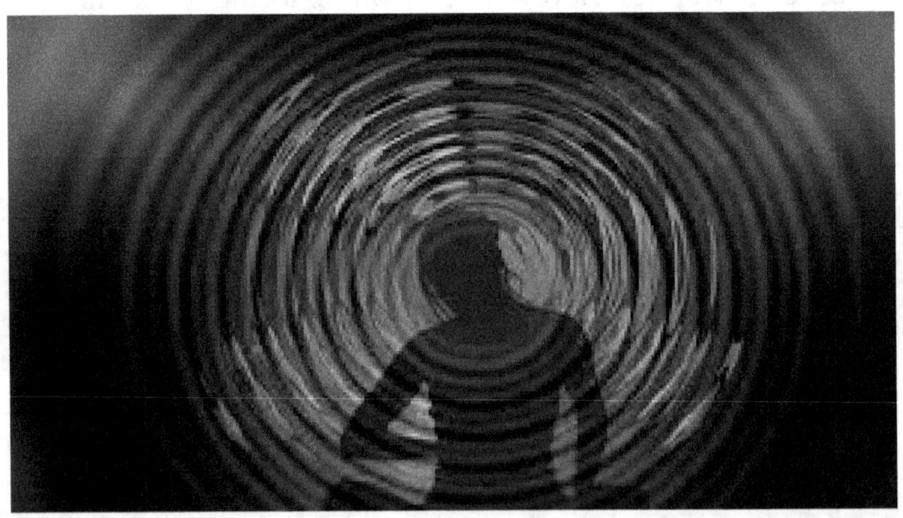

But is there truly energy everywhere? Is the entire world interconnected? If you turned your head right now, you may notice your television, laptop, window, or pet. If you looked outdoors, you might notice some trees, flowers, or your car. Yes, each of these is a distinct entity.

Does this mean that everything is one because everything contains the same material? In actuality, I observe multiple phenomena rather than a single coherent phenomenon.

During your academic career, you may have discovered that molecules make up all matter. You have probably already learned that atoms, which make up all molecules, have nuclei with electrons orbiting around them. These are all parts, fractions, and particles. However, there is no unity or a whole when you first view it. Since appearances might be misleading, it is irrelevant. What appears to be a solid could not be one.

According to scientific evidence, the matter is 99.999999999999 percent space. After the decimal, there are 12 nines. The distance between the first electron and an atom's pinhead-sized nucleus is 160 feet.

There is nothing but space between them. This implies that the majority of this so-called "solid reality"—including what you are reading right now, the object you are sitting on, your home, and the Earth—is empty. There are a lot of open areas there. So, when discussing solid stuff, what is left? You can calculate that the solid portion of an atom makes up only 0.000000000001 percent of the entire atom. It seems unlikely that this tiny amount of solid stuff makes up all solid objects. Everything that appears solid from that perspective is not solid.

Zero Solid Parts

When atoms and molecules were first discovered by scientists in the 1600s, they were thought to be composed of solid objects. There are no "particles" in quantum physics, which was created in the early 1900s. Every aspect of existence is supported by energy. Every particle is thought to vibrate. An electron field will cause electrons to oscillate. The proton field will cause protons to oscillate.

Everything is energy, so everything is interconnected with everything else. The matter won't appear as isolated particles at the most fundamental level. All stuff is an energetically vibrating network of connecting tissues. The majority of space makes up of solid matter and atoms, and this is also true of deep space.

Every beach has the same quantity of sand as there are stars in the entire cosmos. These are endlessly big numbers, but all that space is in between them. That much space is a waste. According to quantum theory, particles have both energy and space between everything. We refer to this as zero-point energy. This validates the adage "Everything is made of energy."

Absolute Energy

Scientists have found that the energy that powers the entire Universe and links everything to everything else in it is not just fundamental energy. Dr. Harold Puthoff conducted the first measurement of this energy. Absolute zero, also known as 0 degrees Kelvin, was used for this experiment. When you boil something by supplying energy to it, the molecules start to move more quickly and quickly. As an illustration, when you heat water, it starts to boil before evaporating. When you freeze water, the reverse takes place. When the water freezes, the molecules start to travel more slowly, causing the water to solidify.

No basic particle, atom, or molecule can move at absolute zero, claims an antiquated scientific theory. This implies that measuring energy should not be possible at this temperature.

He expected to find no energy, but instead, he discovered a surplus of energy that he referred to as "a boiling witch's cauldron."

The Energy of a Thousand Names

The ability of energy to penetrate matter is something that ancient cultures have known for thousands of years but that modern science has just lately discovered. Energy is the source of all things, and energy is the source of all things. All life comes from this source.

It was given a name by every civilization, and this is how it came to be known as "the force with a thousand names." You may be curious as to what this is. It is merely life energy. Since ancient times, every culture has been aware of life force, and they all have a unique term for it. This is known as Chi in Chinese. It is known as pneuma in Greek. In Latin, it is referred to as spiritus Vitalis. In yoga, it is known as prana. The Kahunas of Hawaii refer to it as mana.

It is the Light of the Christian. It is the ka of the ancient Egyptians and the ki of Reiki. In today's society, You will come across this energy in the fluids of mesmerists, the aether of anthroposophy, the od of Reichenback, and the orgone of Wilhelm Reich. In each instance, they are referring to the universal, subtle energy that permeates and encompasses everything. The living force that unites everything is this energy. It creates matter. Life force is frequently used in conjunction with life energy. It has therapeutic and magnetic qualities.

Knowledge and Energy

Every energy field has data in it. This is similar to how performers use scripts to keep themselves organized. This field both influences and absorbs things. It is comparable to incarnation, in which a person's soul assumes a different form. Information functions in the same way. It becomes a form. You require energy to read a book because you have to process the knowledge and then put it into practice.

There is a lot of information created because many individuals equate information and energy. You must understand that energy and information are two distinct properties. Information is provided by a news anchor. We raise the volume if necessary to hear them. You are currently adding energy, but this won't alter the information or the news.

The speaker's information must be communicated to the audience with effort, yet the information will remain the same. If you started speaking louder, no one would suspect that you are telling a different story. You can purchase whatever book you want, but if you don't read it, you won't learn anything from it. Once you've read it, you'll need to invest time and effort into putting what you've learned into practice.

Movements in the Universe

Three processes take place inside of you that are frequently misinterpreted.

The first is your thoughts; the second is your inspirations, and the third is the emotions you experience. Your mind and/or brain produce your thoughts. The vibrations of the universe that you feel deep down but that are largely silent are what inspire you. And the emotions you experience are simply your body's impulses from long ago.

The best gifts you receive from the universe come in the form of feelings, thus you need all three to be functioning properly and being understood appropriately. But we frequently misunderstand them because we think they are the same as the emotions produced by the louder body.

Distinguishing Understanding Inspiration

Are you a meditator? If not, it's time to rethink your entire life plan and approach to achievement. Currently, you may be missing many of the components that will give you a better outcome for the proportionally appropriate level of work if you are not meditating. If you are not meditating, it's also very likely that you are always running two lives: one where you are focused on your goals, and the other where you are constantly cleaning up after failures.

In life, there are two paths to success. You can either receive the answers you need to get on the correct track and accomplish what you need without fighting the repercussions of your failures, or you may let the failure's consequences guide you in the right direction.

Don't misunderstand me. Failure is not a negative thing; in fact, it is the best teacher there is. Its purpose is to reveal to you the mysteries of the cosmos so that you can achieve your goals.

In meditation, experience the universe.

However, meditation employs a different strategy. By preparing you to hear the universe's nudges, meditation ensures that the decisions you make are the right ones. You just, almost instinctively, know what to do in each unique circumstance.

Meditation is the most effective practice someone can perform. Some of you may want to stop practicing meditation if you hold the belief that it is about calmness, Zen, tranquility, prayer, devotion, and spirituality. However, meditation is neither spiritual nor religious. It can be by itself if you so like, yet it is what it is.

As noted in earlier chapters, one way to view meditation is as a force that unifies the opposing systems of the body and mind. The will of the body seems to always move in one direction, whereas the will of the mind seems to always move completely in the opposite direction. We frequently succumb to one or the other, and the guilt we experience is nothing short of debilitating. However, the discussion between the two might be disorganized and upsetting. One result of meditation is that it balances your conflicting systems and unifies the discordant voices. That eliminates noise and creates tranquility throughout.

Have you ever found yourself amid a chaotic argument over whether to pick up a cigarette twelve hours after quitting? The conflict that exists is between your mind, which resolved to quit cold turkey, and your "body," which desires nicotine, or between your mind and your desire to purchase the newest sports car. While one side of you wants to give you the keys, the other side is telling you that the correct move would be to save money and purchase something more affordable.

Each person has experienced many pairs of conflicting forces throughout their life. Sometimes we submit to one force, and other times we triumph over it. Whatever choice we make, the future that results from that choice is influenced by the effects of that choice. Breaking your pledge to stop smoking puts you on a different set of repercussions than not smoking that cigarette. All of us have gone through that.

You can start to realize that there is a third player on the battlefield — sort of a silent umpire — if you look closely at these conflicts and tumultuous disputes. Some refer to it as a conscience, while others refer to it as the soul. But such words come with a lot of baggage that detracts from our topic of achievement and meditation. For the time being, let's call it our core. You must first distinguish between what we refer to as the body and what we refer to as the mind.

We rely on our senses to a large extent to understand the world. We perceive sounds, smells, and so on. None of that is meaningful on its own. Our brain translates what something is and what it signifies from the electrochemical data that our senses alone convey to it. If we have no past introduction to a sense, whether it is sight, hearing, or smell, we will not know what we are seeing or smelling. Through association, we detect non-binary information.

The only two possible outcomes for binary data are one or the other.

On or off, yes or no, correct or incorrect. There aren't any gray areas or in-betweens. The central nervous system could only engage in one of these binary processes initially. But as we developed, our capacity for complex thought and thought patterns increased over a few million years. This way of thinking even enabled us to predict future events using information from the present. The development of the mind and the attitudes that were formed on top of that causes our brain to get more powerful.

We may finally turn consciousness back upon itself and ponder the questions that elevated our being. We could even turn the observation on to ourselves and discover who we are and what we are about. This advanced level of thought is just astonishing.

But behind all of that, at the base of the skull, is the older portion of our brain, which still has some control over decisions under specific conditions. When we encounter the unknown, dread is one of those situations for which we are hard-wired. To keep vigilant against their predators, humans acquired the strong primary emotion of fear. That still affects us now and has the power to alter both the way we think and the results we get.

However, you can transcend the paralyzing quality of fear if you can learn how to access your soul (again, there is no religious reference tied to what is meant by the term soul).

You need to comprehend this book's ultimate goal as we travel through it. Making you the best version of yourself is the theme of this book. Taking control back into your own hands is the theme of this book. It is all about awakening you to the wellspring of your boundless potential and understanding. It aims to demonstrate to you the presence of a teacher you can call upon within. You will receive everything you request if you can look there and ask.

It's not necessary to light candles and close your eyes to meditate. That isn't meditation, though. Silence is not weak; on the contrary, it is one of the most effective tools. If you can access it, you can have whatever you desire, even the greatness you envisage and the power you require.

The road to success is made up of three steps. If you want to advance your skills and transform your life from average to exceptional in one lifetime, you must learn and absorb this way.

The formation and practice of mindfulness are the first steps. The second is the growth of the focus-needed discipline. The many levels of meditation are the last phase.

There is nothing on earth that you cannot accomplish when you set out to do it once you can complete these steps effortlessly.

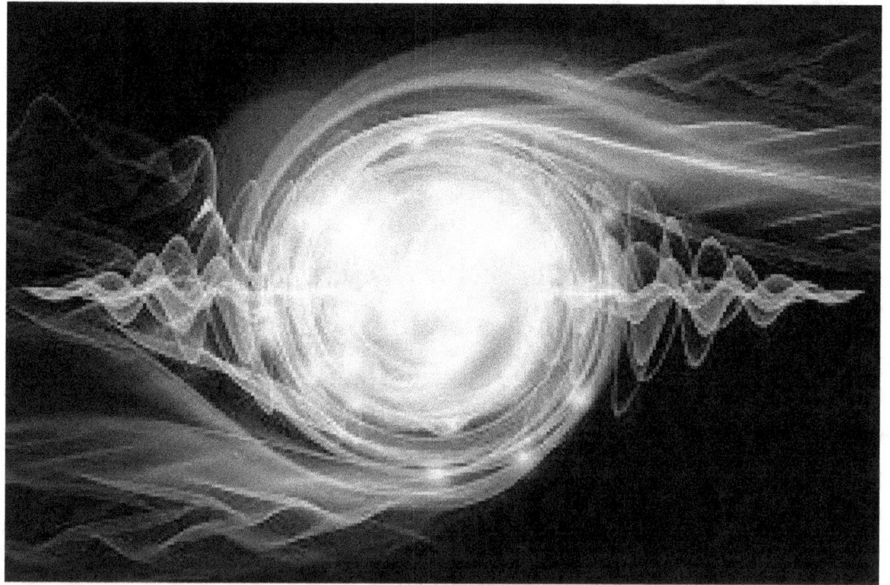

Third Dimension

A typical person can only experience the past, present, and future as realities. He reads its surface-conscious life, but since he cannot see the big picture, he is constrained in what he can achieve. Despite not standing on top of a mountain, he is still a climber. For the higher self, the past and future are figments of the physical mind; all-time modules exist inside the framework of the present. He can withdraw and reflect, predicting the future.

The integration of the past, present, and future inside a frame is the fourth dimension. Because your physical existence will keep you with many perspectives of the past, present, and future until you connect with your higher self, your relationship with that self opens up the fourth dimension.

The fourth dimension resides within us, even though we are physically located in a three-dimensional space. Although it doesn't take physical form, it still has to do with our souls and subconscious minds. Linking the conscious and subconscious minds is required to experience the fourth dimension. It is, to put it simply, the connection between the soul and the reasoning part of the brain. The fourth dimension increases the power of creativity, inspiration, wisdom, and spirituality in a person's life.

The fourth dimension finally reaches a conscious level where you may feel it thanks to a deliberate connection between the brain and the soul that joins the conscious and the subconscious. Conscience is the fourth dimension, which emphasizes the value of welfare, harmony, righteousness, and positivity. Fourth-dimensional thinking enlightens you, helps you actualize your magnificence, and draws you closer to your divine essence.

Those who express their highest form come from a higher consciousness, where they acquire inspiration or original ideas for bringing something into their lives from your higher portion. It frequently presents as an inspiration or an original thought. Inspiration takes with it everyone who needs to reveal energy, vision, clarity, enthusiasm, people, opportunities, resources, and advice when it emanates from their higher selves.

This is why expression requires fourth-dimensional thinking at its core. Everything in your life will materialize by your deepest being when you are manifesting from a higher level of consciousness. The changes that result from broadening one's consciousness and realizing how one's relationship to everything in life works will show up in many different ways.

Advice for triggering the fourth dimension

Beyond our physical existence lies everything in the fourth dimension that has ever existed. You can gain the following skills by adopting a quadrangular mindset:

- ❖ Take on the role of an observer and take in all potential outcomes. Focus on the wider picture.
- ❖ Acquire the skill of effortlessly letting go of the desire for something while holding on to what is already present.
- ❖ Request your best when you want it. • Always pay attention to the core. • Rise above the materialistic mental process and seek the inner light, the meaning of life, and divinity. While your physical mind is always drawn to tangible things, your spirit is always drawn to experiences. Pay close attention to the core of what the item offers.

The sophisticated third-dimensional thinking becomes constrained and senseless as the light of consciousness begins to enter. Anyone can become enraged or upset with the society that disseminated the information.

In the fourth dimension, judgments still take place but are far less tactile. In every situation, spirituality is the topic.

This needs a conscience that has awakened.

Vibration Pattern

Because you are formed of matter, and we all know that matter is the vibrating state of energy, every part of you, from the tissue of your beating heart to the tips of your fingernails, vibrates in a certain way.

Force and matter can be created from energy. You already know that momentum, which is force, is a property of matter and may be used to move it. Picture ice floating in a body of water. The ice may be moved by the water, and both substances are identical at various vibrational frequencies.

Every live and inanimate entity, from humans to thoughts, from planets to space, is bound together by a fabric that lies underneath space and time. Ancient meditation masters have known it to exist, and science has recently verified this. They are known as fields in science, and each fundamental particle has a unique field. The elements that makeup matter are created by a vibration in that field. The Swiss Large Hadron Collider is being tested not to identify particles but to discover the fields that produce these particles.

And they have achieved great success.

You must have realized by this point that you are an object that vibrates continuously. similar to a tuning fork. You are related to everything else in the universe consisting of energy and matter through the field that vibrates to create you. As closely related to your twin as rock salt buried in the Himalayas is to you.

The Law of Attraction operates on the premise that everything is connected to everything else and that everything is what it is because of its unique vibrational signature.

Your frequency serves as the foundation for all you do and who you develop into from birth to death. But it's not entirely self-sufficient. It requires your involvement to receive direction. Consider an automobile descending a slope. Whatever your stance, it will continue.

It will reach the incline's base. You can direct the direction the car goes if you take the wheel. Without realizing it, you will unconsciously draw all kinds of things into your life. Controlling where you receive the effects of this power is the thing you need to do. Whatever you do, you always vibrate at a certain frequency. But there are several ways you may manage it. One approach to managing your vibration is through exercise. Another one is meditation. While meditation, sleep, and classical music (such as Bach, Vivaldi, and Tessarini) will all reduce your vibration, exercise, dancing, and techno music will all raise it.

Walking is another way to change your vibrational profile. You have a vibrational profile that you are born with; this vibration manifests as you, but you can move that vibration in any of the ways that have been mentioned. Each person must discover the method that best controls their vibration. A decent rule of thumb is to consider body type while choosing the right activity for a person to manage his vibration.

What Your Vibration Profile Is

There are three different forms of vibrational bodies. The first is the person who, despite eating well, never seems to gain weight.

These people have a lot of energy and are quite highly strung. If this describes you, learning to practice mindful meditation is the best approach to controlling your vibration. You should lower the tuning.

The greatest technique to change your vibrational energy if you are the overweight kind that finds it difficult to lose weight and has highly oily skin is to engage in vigorous activity at least once per day, followed by deep breathing exercises. Increase your vibrational profile, then.

You are the one who falls into the third body type and is neither of the first two. The greatest workout for you to do to get your vibration in order is to eat frequently, whenever you are hungry, get lots of fresh air, and meditate. These activities will get your vibration into the desired range and get you to the location where you need to be to regulate that frequency. Avoid consuming caffeine. You must be able to control your vibrational swings to prevent them from becoming excessively high or low for this body type.

Whatever your body type, meditation will always be beneficial.

You can always benefit from combining introspection, mindfulness, and meditation to raise your vibrational frequency.

The various regimens for achieving optimal vibration are founded on straightforward logic. Different bodily types function at various vibrational levels. The more active a person is, the higher their vibration, and as a result, they have stronger metabolisms and don't seem to put on weight as quickly. Low energy types are a little heavier since they have slower metabolisms.

Once you know what type of body you have, you can start experimenting with different workout frequencies and balancing them with meditation to discover your ideal vibration. It will be to your advantage if you practice yoga.

Because you may use meditation techniques to raise your vibration, meditation and mindfulness are effective for all body types. When you're at peace, you've attained the vibration that works best.

Without the practitioner trying to determine whether they need to raise or lower their vibration, meditation automatically creates a feeling of tranquility by raising or reducing energy.

It's all about the vibration, so keep that in mind. Once you develop the habit of vibrating at the proper frequency, using the Law of Attraction's cutting edge will come naturally as a result of your efforts.

Getting in tune with the Universe's Vibration

For the LOA to be effective for you, you must become attuned to the vibration of the universe. Your physical energy is increased, which enhances your cerebral and verbal output. The key to raising your vibration is improving how you feel about yourself.

Since happiness is the goal of life, you should schedule regular time for self-happiness. There are several angles from which to view this.

In general, you always want to be where your vibration is at its highest, which is when you're in a good mood. It's pretty much the best spot to be in life to be happy. When you're in a good mood, things normally run well around you and you're willing to go with the flow. The only issue with that is that it's challenging to always be cheerful, so we have to work at it.

Your vibration will increase as your mood improves. It's likely that you already know what makes you happy. excellent music, working out, meditating, taking a stroll, etc.

Nevertheless, some approaches are superior to others for maximizing the usage of the LOA.

Without a doubt, dancing is the finest way to enhance your vibration.

Your body may relax and your mind can unite with your body while listening to engaging music and moving your body. Physical exercise can cause the mind and body to become one, allowing you to enter a thoughtless but emotionally rich state of mind. similar to the runner's high.

Take advantage of the opportunity to listen to your favorite music while driving; music that gets your heart pumping. Additionally, if you were already experiencing your "end" result, dancing is one of those things you might engage in more frequently.

The best moment to employ affirmations is when you're in this mindset, or even better when you're speaking them aloud.

Just picture a group of Native Americans chanting and dancing in front of a fire.

To raise their energy and more quickly access what they are attempting to do, they are producing a charge of energy. Another illustration is the Turkish whirling dervishes; this particular dancing style induces a state of heightened awareness that can result in a profoundly joyful state of being, or this case, a deeper relationship with God.

If you practice martial arts, you may have noticed that some styles are centered on the yin and yang principle, which involves body movements that seamlessly transition into one another in a very rhythmic way, much as you would when dancing. Traditional martial arts are based on the body's organic movements. Because of this, some martial art artists can make little movements with such strength, like Bruce Lee's one-inch punch. He had a complete understanding of how the body worked, and he mentally merged with it.

Things to Remember

The first step in achieving a goal is to set one; a goal is a target. Spend some time and give every aspect of the goal you want to create careful thought. If you are just getting started with the LOA, you need a goal that is at least somewhat attainable.

Always aim higher after you've hit your target. You visualize, meditate, and pay daily attention to achieving a significant goal.

The minor goals develop from the major goal and serve as the necessary steps to achieve the overall aim. Take the modest measures that will help you get to "the ultimate result" every day.

The importance of daily meditation or setting aside time to focus on the desired outcome cannot be overstated. Losing sight of your objective signals a lack of commitment to accomplishing it. If that's the case, it's alright, but you need to choose a goal that motivates you and can help you realize a deeper purpose.

Like an Olympic athlete, you must take daily action for your goal to materialize. It is worthwhile to set aside 15 minutes each day for meditation. If you think that will take too much time, you may not understand the value of focus or the influence your subconscious mind has over your conscious consciousness. Spending time concentrating is like fine-tuning a tool that directs you toward the target, in this instance your brain.

You can recognize your true desires for life by spending time with yourself. Spending time alone illuminates what it is to be human and increases your capacity for empathy and relatability. We all have similar minds, so understanding how your function can help you understand how others think.

Finding strategies to particularly elevate your vibration when you're by yourself can be beneficial. Workouts, strolls, beautiful music, and dancing all allow a deeper understanding to seep through to your conscious consciousness. While using visualization or affirmations, raising your vibration likewise raises the vibration of those concepts.

The secret to starting a new life is developing new habits of feeling and thinking. You are surrounded by things that were once believed and thought to be true. Regardless of your surroundings, you must constantly be and consider the change you want to see in the world right now. Be innovative and transformative.

Exercise 1:

List five things you can do to assist in the expansion of your company.

Use the following inquiries as a starting point.

- ❖ Do you have network access?
- ❖ Can you ask your coworkers what they did to expand their businesses?
- ❖ Possess you a website?
- ❖ Should your website be updated?
- ❖ Is your office in need of an update?
- ❖ Can you pick up a new talent?
- ❖ Should you hire someone?
- ❖ Are you able to carry that out?
- ❖ Make a list and complete every item on it.

Exercise 2:

Spend some time every day practicing one or more of the different meditation techniques. Focus on the one that feels most comfortable for you. The optimum times to imagine your "end" goal and speak affirmations are in the morning and at night.

An excellent time to observe your thoughts is after you have completely awakened.

To learn to separate yourself from your ideas, you might require more mental strength.

Exercise 3: Throughout the day, spend five minutes periodically refocusing on your vision.

Learn to remove yourself from stressful situations that dominate your thoughts, and use your emotions as a guide to comprehend these situations.

Exercise 4: Don't put off the things you want to do; spend some of your free time doing them because life is shorter than you think. Try to engage in actions that will make you feel as though you have already achieved the desired outcome, and as you accomplish them, try to feel appreciation or thanks for it.

Mindfulness

The discipline and practice of mindfulness have been extensively studied in the literature. Additionally, there is an awful misunderstanding of what mindfulness is, which is even more prevalent than the unfortunate misunderstanding of what meditation is.

To apply mindfulness as a precursor to meditation, you must be aware of three things. The first is that mindfulness involves planning your time and space. The second is that mindfulness is about bringing your conscious mind into sync with where you are in time and space right now.

Finally, practicing mindfulness involves developing your conscious ability, which starts little and can grow to have immense strength.

For you to comprehend the scale of your mindfulness and how it relates to the entirety of the universe, we shall expose you to two cosmic phenomena.

Two measurements of an environment found throughout the cosmos are space and time. The dimensions of space and time vanish beyond the edge of the cosmos. Matter and everything that results from the existence of matter is created by the same energy that establishes the boundaries of this space and time.

Time and space are both more than what a ruler and a clock can capture. We are aware that time is a unique phenomenon that is not uniform throughout space, contrary to what Einstein postulated and what physicists have since demonstrated.

Except to suggest that we need to view time as a stream, going too deeply into the physics and intricacies of time would not make much sense. Although there are many applications for the analogy being used right now, caution should be exercised when using it. Beyond this, it serves a purpose, but it could be ineffective.

We consider time to be a stream because it moves in only one direction, which is crucial for maintaining mindfulness.

Second, depending on how vast your conscious mind may be, you can see time as wide as a river or as narrow as a stream. The last reason the river analogy is effective is that it enables you to view events that take place across space as passing through time, much like a river.

Being present in both space and time

Numerous activities are taking place all around us. Imagine being able to view everything happening in the universe right now, from a fry hatching to the birth of the sun in a far-off region of the cosmos. That's a lot of data streams — a river that's quite vast.

Consider, though, if you only had one screen and that screen displayed your breathing. The movement of air in and out of you is the only thing, and as far as you are concerned, the entire universe is reduced to this one act. The second symbolizes a fairly narrow river, while the first resembles an indefinitely wide river with a lot of data. If you're given a vast river to manage but only can comprehend and control one stream, your mind will crash. You feel overpowered and unable to comprehend your surroundings.

The issue with feeling overwhelmed is that your brain's circuit breakers fail as soon as you do, making it impossible for you to process your surroundings and whatever is in front of you. That emotion is all too familiar to us. When you are unable to comprehend your surroundings, fear — a primal emotion — takes control. Because of how we are wired, we naturally fear the unknown. When you are feeling overpowered, you will experience fear. For some people, this might even trigger anxiety and panic episodes.

You may slow down the flow of information and lessen the sense of overload by practicing mindfulness. As most people online would claim, practicing mindfulness involves more than just concentrating on one thing at a time.

Being mindful means concentrating only on what your stream of consciousness allows. The majority of people begin by doing one item at a time. You may do the same, and after practicing for a while, you'll discover that you can multitask by only doing one item at a time.

Your thoughts and actions must be cogently related.

The most important aspect of this is that the present should be your point of emphasis. Never should the discussion center on either the past or the future. Additionally, because you can only be in one place at a time, you will naturally concentrate on the location and time of that location. When you do that, your stream's entire width is applied to that one point.

When you focus your concentration on one item, rather than moving forward or backward in time, you can look at that one thing more thoroughly than just its outward features. As your mindfulness skills advance, you'll discover that you can explore the object of your attention more deeply and comprehend it viscerally.

You will strengthen or, in this example, expand that stream as much as you exercise it. You can apply more of yourself to the present than before when you enlarge that stream. You will keep seeing things you couldn't see before as this keeps expanding.

Your stream's size will never be the same as another person's. At the same moment, some people can process more in their conscious mind than others. You begin to increase that when you engage in mindfulness practice.

It is really easy to get started with mindfulness. This may be accomplished practically anywhere using any method. After all, practicing mindfulness simply entails doing and thinking simultaneously while delving more deeply into the processes involved. However, if you insist on being more rigorous about it, take a seat on a cozy chair. Focus on the air that enters and leaves your nose by closing your eyes to eliminate visual distractions. You may restore order to chaos by using your breath as a natural metronome. It is customary to do this, therefore you ought to feel at ease carrying it out.

Allow your body to do what it does best; do not attempt to regulate the rate at which you breathe. All you have to do is relax and watch. Sit back and count it if you find it difficult to watch. One for entry and one for the exit. Count on till you reach ten, then begin again. When you're comfortable with it, you can stop counting and focus just on your breathing.

When you can complete the brief sessions, it's time to develop new skills. Taking the sessions out of your sofa and into the real world is the next stage. From the moment you wake up until the moment you go to bed, you can practice mindfulness in all of your activities. You will discover that you can complete tasks more quickly and precisely if you can apply the breathing technique to them.

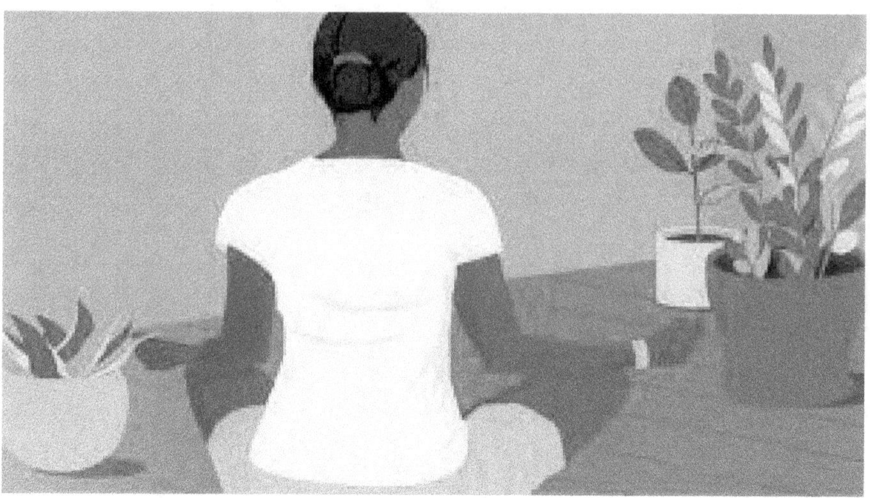

By this time, mindfulness will come effortlessly to you, and you'll be surprised by how much more you take in throughout each waking hour. Additionally, you'll discover that you don't even need to take notes during meetings because you can remember everything by simply paying attention to the people you listen to. You'll discover that you can recall people's names and faces. Your ability would significantly rise.

You should continue to practice being attentive every day on your own even after you master it. Despite being utilized as a gateway to meditation, mindfulness is not meditation. However, it is a discipline that you employ to hone other faculties of your mind and soul.

Practices for Mindfulness

You can utilize three exercises to improve and sustain your capacity for mindfulness. Even if you complete mindful training and master successful meditation, there will still be days when you require additional support. There will be a time when you are unable to concentrate or meditate. When it happens, these workouts will be beneficial.

First-stage breathing This has already been discussed, and it should be sufficient to get you started. However, there is another technique to employ breathing to increase your sense of awareness.

For this, you can be anywhere. It makes no difference if you're in a coffee shop or on a train. It's up to you whether you keep your eyes open or shut for this. Start by taking a deep breath in, pause, and then exhale slowly and deliberately. Do this three times, focusing intently each time on the point of your nose where it meets the bridge of your forehead. Consider observing that location. It almost appears as though you have crossed your eyes if your eyes are open.

Complete three sets of deep inhalations while gazing at that location, then, with your eyes closed, resume regular breathing. Up to ten breaths per count. then reset to zero once more. Repeat the count up to 9. then reset to 0 again. Once more count up to 8. Then it returns to zero. If you get off course, start over at number 10 immediately. Each person is different, so you shouldn't speed up or slow down to stay inside this time. This should take you approximately five minutes. Take it easy and move at your own pace.

You will be surprised to see that your attitude changes while you work, and finally your perspective on things become new when you finish and open your eyes. While you may be inclined to absorb everything, strive to focus your attention on the things that need it most.

Most successful businesspeople who do this immediately start working on projects that use their creative abilities. Or they do it before exercising.

Stage 2

The next level you can try is somewhat less challenging but calls for downloading an app on your smartphone. Alternatively, you could just set a minute-by-minute recurring alert. A bell will sound during this exercise at predetermined intervals. My phone gently chimes every twenty minutes for me. My magic interval is twenty minutes, and that appears to be effective for me. That will undoubtedly change over time.

Due to my natural window of efficiency, 20 minutes has been my thing. It generally only takes me 20 minutes to complete anything. And right now, I'm making sure that one of two things is the focus of my renewed and updated attention. Sometimes, I have to move on to the next assignment because it's time to do so. Or I should breathe in and focus more intently on the same activity.

This has been quite helpful to me in increasing my productivity. Although many of us who practice this have discovered that there is no correlation between our effective windows, one thing has remained constant: everyone is unique.

The alarm now starts to sound. Take three long, cleansing breaths while closing your eyes. Once it's finished, return to your primary task.

Stage 3 This stage calls for you to pick up a new skill. At this point, you start integrating awareness into every aspect of your life. not only each evening or hour. This is done to encourage you to spend your time fully, not in one spot while your feet are elsewhere.

Your location must match where your thoughts are. Both making plans and pondering how something might turn out are not seen as going against this.

All of these mental paths are free will choices. The important thing is that you are just thinking about what you are doing right now.

By making stage one and stage two simple to complete, you achieve this. That requires effort over time. You must be diligent to make sure that these actions become habits. It's helpful to be able to develop habits, but habits aren't about carrying out tasks automatically; instead, they serve to remind you of what needs to be done and when.

You start your day by telling yourself that you'll maintain a level of mindful focus throughout the entire day (the focus part will come later).

You tell yourself that this is the way to success and that it will have the biggest impact with the least amount of work. From that point forward, you must be ruthless and vigilant at all times.

Making you docile like a rabbit on your way to mindfulness and meditation is not the goal. It's designed to make you as fierce as a lion.

Nothing about this mindfulness practice or meditation is meant to give you the impression that you are about to become submissive and kind. It's not. You need to awaken the lion within you so that you can focus on one goal and achieve it. Successes are created in this manner.

Get yourself back to your destination if you see that you are veering off course. To do it, use the breathing exercise. If you discover that you are easily distracted, perform a quick exercise to expend the excess energy and increase circulation before concentrating on the labored breathing. Keep your composure and concentrate on it as the intensity increases. Once it starts working for you, you'll come to cherish this kind of energized calm.

internal fortitude

Have you ever realized that similar to other people, you possess a wealth of positive traits within yourself?

Most of us have no idea how we have such hidden talents.

What's left of us don't have the slightest idea how to remove the traits from any discernible block and use them to improve an incredible concept or in driving a more rewarding background, regardless of whether we are aware that they are present inside of us. Permit us to investigate methods and strategies to expose our hidden traits to enhance our life.

In any event, you ought to think of yourself as possessing some unusual qualities.

Stop self-critical thoughts.

Never say "I can't" to yourself. Instead, visualize yourself with the necessary traits to combat any condition, regardless of what it may be, and know that, if you do it correctly, you can and will unquestionably prevail.

Keep in mind that self-conviction is assurance, and gaining certainty is a significant portion of the struggle.

The next step is to begin your self-exploration. Nearly look into your experience and genetics. Not that you haven't already done this.

could have. You will gradually need to perform it even more effectively. Note the gifts you received from your family or grandparents. If you don't believe you have any, consider what they have told you.

Is it conceivable that you possess such wonderful traits somewhere deep within you? You haven't realized that you could employ them, in any case. enumerate all the traits and skills of your ancestors or grandparents.

Check to see if any or all of them can be used.

Does music, for instance, still run in the family?

Have you ever noticed how stable your mother was in such large doses?

Additionally, you could model it without actually doing it.

Have you ever noticed that you fundamentally speak in a way that people you know don't? Have you not made amazing use of this bent? Perhaps you have a strong body to contribute.

However, you don't consider the practices that could make the best use of your physical attributes. Investigate, try, and then abuse. Your framework for removing your qualities from any limiting impact should be that.

Focus on Your Personal Qualities

You feel that your newly acquired establishment is becoming easier for you to understand. In any case, you require a thorough evaluation. Prepare another unambiguous statement of the qualities your planning and guidance have given you.

What range of abilities do you possess?

Is it true that you are making the best use of your skills and qualities?

Have you considered your interests, converted some of them into side pursuits, and considered the possibility of developing at least one of the latter into a future profession?

List your inner strengths for achieving success in your life, such as restraint, compassion, negotiation, watchfulness, constancy, confirmation, etc.

This exercise is not unique in any way. Periodic evaluations of your traits will enable you to identify subtle traits that might point you in the appropriate direction as your life progresses. You never know; you might get lucky!

Alternating Observations

Enhance your personality and traits while structuring, and decide how to respond to situations in the world both verbally and non-verbally. Let's start by acknowledging that your perception of reality is based on subjectivity.

What you perceive to be true is merely a concealed description of this current reality, not just truth, just as a guide is only a less than a typical description of a location. The desire to see everything through rosy-colored lenses is something you can't resist. Your responses are controlled less by reality than by how you see it.

Neuro-linguistic programming, often known as NLP, helps you understand this and minimizes, if not eliminates, your subjectivity. At that moment, you can consider choosing your perspectives on the current situation to decide on how to respond to it.

Why do people respond differently to a particular event or condition? Is it not due to their limitations in terms of how they perceive that circumstance or event? One person's awful setback may not be the same as another's.

For instance, some individuals may take offense or choose to disregard verbal or physical abuse. Others may be so negatively impacted that they need mental health therapy.

NLP's core philosophy is centered on the idea that one may alter their perception, feelings, and behavior to justify terrifying situations. You might even become immune to harm.

The most frequent barrier to achieving our goals is that we frequently base our emotions on how we see our current situation. For instance, we frequently seek abundance because we have already encountered the reverse. We declare that we want abundance, yet when it comes to our financial situation or bank account balance, we get frustrated and concentrate on the scarcity of abundance.

We feel anxious and unhappy as a result of what we observe. By doing this, we unintentionally adopt a mindset of scarcity (the antithesis of abundance) and draw more instances of financial hardship into our lives. Then, as we consider those conditions, we continue to feel bad about being broke.

The cycle continues.

Understanding that we need to place more emphasis on what we want rather than what it is is crucial if we want to stop this cycle. Regardless matter what we are currently seeing, we must find ways to think and feel abundantly if we want abundance. The idea of money is not always useful in situations like this. Numerous negative emotions and beliefs are associated with money, some of which we developed as young children.

We assume and absorb these beliefs when our parents tell us things like, "We cannot afford it," "Money doesn't grow on trees," or "You were not born rich like so-and-so," and they remain buried deep in our subconscious for years to come.

Then, we frequently unconsciously believe that we don't deserve financial prosperity, that we aren't deserving of it, and that we aren't deserving of luck, youth, or intelligence to have it.

Keep in mind that most of this is subconscious, so even though you may say, "Of course I know I deserve it!" in your head, your subconscious holds a belief that is contrary to that: it holds the notion that it is more powerful and will undermine your conscious attempts. Therefore, it is crucial to reprogram the subconscious mind, yet it may also be advantageous to completely avoid talking about money.

It's an amazing aim to say you want to be a millionaire, but if you're not there yet or have never been, it could be hard for you to consciously believe it. How do you picture such a goal, furthermore? Limiting oneself to merely seeing bank account balances or mountains of cash might be difficult.

Go more broadly and leave the topic of money alone. Think about hoping for abundance and freedom rather than wishing to become a millionaire. Consider all the things you would do with the money rather than specific dollar quantities. Where do you want to reside? What design would you choose for your home? Which would you purchase? How about a destination?

Who would you assist? Immerse yourself in those thoughts and emotions. What would you think about it? Relieved? Free?

Appreciating? Grateful? Abundant? These are all the vibrations you need to be to fulfill your objectives. Because your mind cannot tell the difference between reality and imagination, when you think and feel wealthy thoughts and emotions, you are essentially retraining your mind to be in a wealthy state of being.

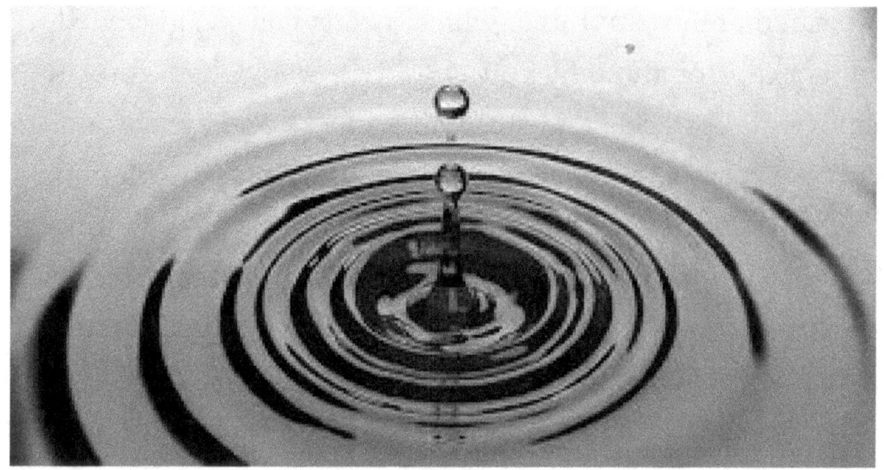

Manifesting

You can manifest anything, which means you can give life to any concept or thought you choose. If and when you can remove all obstacles and stumbling blocks and synchronize with the cosmos, wishes do come true. If you pay attention to what occurs to you and those around you, you will notice that the Law of Manifestation that you need to understand is present everywhere. You already know it to be true; all I need to do is show you how to put it into action.

You still have to exercise. To receive something in this material realm is to manifest it. It is a present. It is a blessing, and you should be thankful for it, regardless of how diligently and intelligently you worked for it. You'll receive more as soon as you are. Once you have more, you must share it with people who don't know how to obtain it rather than giving it to them without charge. Teach them how to fish instead of giving them the fish. After receiving so much, one of the ways I give back is by teaching you how to do it. I can assure you that if you give more, you will receive more.

We have covered significant territory in this book. To help you comprehend that there is a logical explanation for all of this, we started at the fundamental question and looked at the structure of the universe. By this point, you ought to be able to see that turning your dreams into reality requires more than one step. It's not even a task that can be completed in stages.

This is not a pudding recipe.

To live the life of a conduit who can ask the universe for anything they need and have it flow through them into reality, you must adopt a lifestyle that synchronizes all these abilities. similar to how Thomas Edison brought forth the light bulb.

It seems sensible to inquire as to how one manifests. However, after reading this book, trying to figure out how to materialize is like trying to teach a tuning fork how to play a note. You might occasionally be able to realize your dreams if you follow a list, but it's more likely that you won't. However, if you alter your perspective, adjust your vibration, and proceed with caution in life, you will be able to attract anything you desire.

Because of the following three events: You can first find inspiration for the things you want. That implies that your desires won't be arbitrary or passing fancies. You'll begin to recognize your genuine worth and the things that are important to you. When this occurs, you'll start manifesting more easily.

Second, because you will have the strength to push anything out of your way and climb over obstacles that would often trip anyone else, you will start to have the energy to take the action required to make things happen.

Finally, you'll be able to always produce the ideal vibration.

When you reach this level, things will come to you automatically in addition to being able to manifest frequently. They'll be standing in front of you, ready and waiting for you.

Making your desires come true and creating a purposeful, goal-based life are both aspects of manifesting.

I have some extra remarks for those of you asking how to manifest the new Porsche or the new Gulfstream 650. Rewards vs. Achievement

There is nothing wrong with valuing comfort and financial gain. When you are inspired by the fruits of your success, there is nothing wrong with that. Don't feel bad about it or like a bad person for enjoying the perks of a prosperous life.

However, this book has more to offer than that.

Anyone with good credit will be able to obtain a loan to purchase a Ferrari. Gulfstream has financed. Or you could even own a jet timeshare. What's so special about that? The accomplishment is what you should concentrate on because the reward will always come after. You are merely picturing the benefits you seek when you picture the sports car in your driveway or the superyacht in the harbor.

However, if you concentrate your abilities of manifestation on earning $1,000,000 per day, $10,000,000 per day, or even $100,000,000 per day, you will end up producing the vibration that leads to power. You can easily purchase the toys you desire with 100 million a day.

Another thing is if you ask for something like a yacht and concentrate on the reward. the events that follow receiving the yacht. What happens if you only manage to scrounge together a loan when the yacht is docked? Next, what? There will be a big disappointment.

You should aspire to success instead. The benefits will come after.

I'd want to leave you with one final thing to think about. The universe only provides for your needs, which could include obstacles. Bad things are exactly what you will manifest if you wish for them. You will manifest negativity if you are negative and vibe negatively. Even disasters are manifestable. This is why people who have negative beliefs experience unpleasant occurrences, which only serves to strengthen their belief that bad things always do.

You need to start thinking positively if you experience a lot of negative events in your life. Reread Chapter 4 to review the abilities you must develop to think positively and begin making changes in your life. You can discover that you can have good in your life and it can be good after good with only one occurrence that you positively seek, believe you deserve and let happen without hesitation. It is what you anticipate will occur.

Energy is the source from which everything manifests. What we think of as separate and solid is an illusion. A continuously moving, interconnected sphere of energy that vibrates at various frequencies lies beneath it.

Quantum energy fields that are vibrating at a specific frequency and interacting in specific ways make up solid matter.

Although matter may seem to be solid, it vibrates and moves constantly at the subatomic level. Even though they vibrate at much higher frequencies and interact with the surrounding field of energies, thoughts, and emotions are forms of energy. The frequency of thought of love or joy is entirely different from that of thought of hopelessness or rage.

Positive thoughts of a certain frequency will attract more energy of that frequency to them because energy attracts more of its kind (positive events). Equally unpleasant thoughts will likewise draw like frequencies, causing compulsive negative thinking and associated occurrences to become aware.

You have a physical experience, yet you are an energy being. We are vibration translators in our physical bodies; using our senses, we decipher various frequencies. You are energy, and when you put out a signal at a certain frequency, you draw other frequencies of the same frequency back to you. Although thoughts and feelings are high-frequency energies that the senses cannot perceive, they nonetheless exist. Your thoughts and feelings control the frequency you emit and therefore attract.

The Emotional Handbook

You can use your emotions as a lovely and useful guide on your path to creation. Positive emotions indicate that you are moving in the right direction to achieve your goals. You are of course if you are having bad feelings. How you feel makes it simple to identify what you are concentrating on. Your emotions are boosted and you feel happy, joyous, and excited if your vibration matches what you want. The frequency will typically be lower when you are concentrating on shortage, which will cause lower emotions like worry, anxiety, irritation, or hopelessness.

Your most frequent thoughts and emotions are reflected in your present physical reality.

Since the majority of us have not yet mastered the ability to actively regulate and direct our emotions, this may initially seem overwhelming. The good news is that you can always select how you want to feel, making this one of your most useful tools. You may not be able to influence the feelings or behaviors of other people, but you can always manage your feelings and ideas. Simply thinking about anything positive, whether it is already a part of your life or is something you want it to be, will help you feel more positive or high vibrational.

Being able to retain inner calm, joy, and contentment despite external situations is what defines true freedom. And you may accomplish this by repeatedly picking a concept that makes you feel better, regardless of what is happening around you.

For you to manifest your wants, your beliefs must also vibrate at the same frequency. You cannot desire something, concentrate on its absence, and then hope to obtain it since they are two very distinct frequencies. You must tune into its frequency to receive it.

Be mindful of the factors that you let shape your experience.

The media and the news can cause a lot of unpleasant ideas and sensations, so paying too much attention to them might lower your energy. Always strive for your best emotions. It is much preferable to watch shows that make you laugh and feel good overall than ones that cause fear or anxiety.

In a similar vein, pay attention to who you spend time with and how you communicate with them. Do those nearby regularly voice complaints? Do they frequently discuss their issues? Do they judge or engage in gossip? All of these are detrimental factors that have to be maintained to a minimum. Make a conscious effort to avoid these types of conversations whenever possible because they cause you to vibrate at a lower frequency and are therefore more likely to trigger unpleasant emotions.

Do you frequently vent to others about your problems? If this applies to you, make an effort to stop engaging in this kind of conduct. Complaining or sharing your unpleasant situations with others just serves to keep the issue going. You practically relive and revitalize it as you talk about it again and over. You also concentrate on it, which causes you to experience the accompanying emotions and thoughts. As a result, your energy aligns with that of your issue, which keeps bringing more of it into your experience.

Avert comparing yourself to others. This is an utterly worthless mental exercise that rarely enhances your experience in any way.

Everybody's journey is unique and personal. Just concentrate on your own experience and your capacity to influence it in the direction you desire. Only your world and experiences are under your control.

Why do we seek prosperity? We do it because we think it would improve our mood. Everything we desire in life is a result of our conviction that it will somehow improve our mood. Knowing that you always have a choice in how you feel will help you feel better now. You will then fulfill your desire by giving this frequency. As a result, the only manifestation you should strive for is the sensation of your desire.

Your desired emotion will materialize. You may do this anytime, anyplace, as long as you concentrate on creating the sensation and feeling of what you like. Make achieving that your main goal and the physical will catch up.

By observing how you feel, you can quickly determine where you are in the emotional spectrum (figure below). This vibe is what you are presently giving forth. You begin climbing up this range by aiming for a better feeling notion. You'll feel some alleviation or a modest improvement as a result. Keep in mind that you cannot get from despair to joy immediately. It is impossible to achieve this significant vibrational difference. By aiming for emotion with a higher frequency, experiencing relief, gaining stability, and then climbing up again, you steadily rise the emotional scale.

How to Clear Manifestations

We must be clear to attract what we desire. The brain receives 11 million pieces of information per second. Only 15 bits of information are processed by us each second. What about the remaining 10.999985 pieces of data? The brain just filters those out as being unimportant to our existence. Everybody's analysis is unique.

Therefore, if we can alter the filter that evaluates all incoming data, we can alter how it is processed, allowing the filter to accept additional information or even more. To interact with our subconscious mind at this point, we must first become clear.

Limiting ideas that have been pre-programmed into our subconscious minds are overburdened by life experiences and, in some cases, genetic information about the experiences of our ancestors and relatives. Let's use the desire for financial wealth as an example. But nothing is taking place. Money is the source of all evil is a saying that may be operating in your subconscious, yet this is a limiting concept that we have all heard at some point in our lives. We are prevented from accomplishing our goals by the restrictive assumption that we will never have enough money. This constricting idea needs to be dispelled.

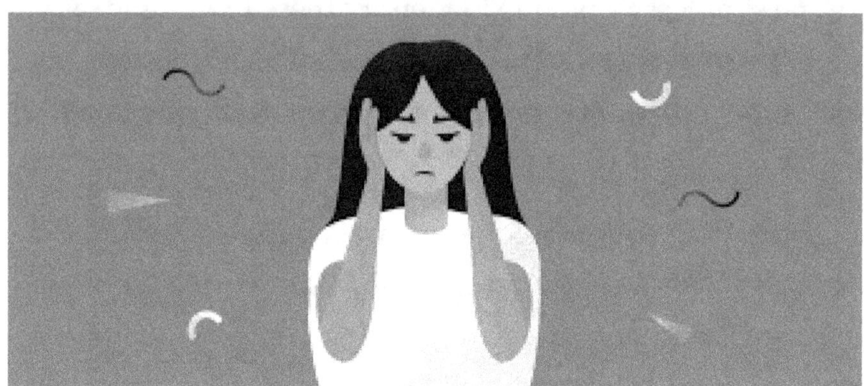

Determine your limiting assumptions.

How can I identify my limiting beliefs? That is the key question since without knowing what to clear, we can't begin. Or we can, but it will be simpler for us to get rid of them if we know what they are.

The simplest technique to identify these limiting ideas is to sit in meditation and picture what you desire. For example, if you want a pricey car, picture it in your mind's eye.

Then, you could become aware of the thoughts and emotions that are coming to you. Are you angry and depressed? Perhaps you're thinking, "I'll never have the money to buy that automobile," "What would my father say if I had a better car than him," or "I don't deserve that kind of car." Write them down because they represent the limiting ideas that prevent you from owning that car.

You wish to be a skilled public speaker, for instance. Sit and picture yourself giving a speech in front of others. When you have anxiety, explore it and see what comes up for you. Is your fear of public speaking a result of a previous experience? Do you want what happened in the past to have an impact on you now? Can I let that go instead? You might think, "I can't do it, I'm too scared, I stutter and flush," or anything like that. You can now identify and eliminate your limiting beliefs from your life.

What is clearing? There are numerous techniques for eradicating limiting beliefs; in this book, we'll discuss four of them: thankfulness in the present, EFT, the "Do I believe that" technique, and Ho'oponopono.

In the present, gratitude

There may not be a simpler way to clear it than this. The secret is to be grateful for everything you have in life, whether it's a pen, a child, a house, or a flower. Simply feel thankful right now, in your current location. Your day will only grow better if you get off to a good start. Therefore, whenever something bothers you or you have a negative emotion that you don't want to have or that you believe is out of character for the circumstance, utilize this skill and express thankfulness for something in your life to prevent the negative emotion from controlling you. For instance, when you receive distressing news, you could feel a lump in your throat. Just notice the feeling; don't ignore it; just feel it; and then, in your mind, focus on something for which you are grateful. The change will be very strong.

EFT stands for emotional freedom technique. Because it is one of the most effective methods for releasing the tension, life coaches frequently employ this. The method incorporates tapping and particular affirmations.

At a certain location on the body, tapping is done with the tips of the fingers.

Decide on a scale of one to ten how strong the negative emotion is before you start tapping. When you're finished, you can evaluate it once again to determine how well it affected that particular emotion.

First, while saying, "Even though I have this blah blah (fill in the problem you have a limiting belief, bad feeling, or something else), I sincerely and completely accept myself," tap on the outside of your hand. As an illustration, the crucial stage is to acknowledge how this situation affects your feelings. While tapping the first tapping spot, you repeat these three times (outside the hand). When pressing the other places, you don't have to utter the entire statement; instead, you might say things like "This limiting belief" "That money is terrible," "This hurting shoulder," or "This fear of spiders."

1) the outside of the hand is the first tapping point (karate chop)
2) browse (both sides)
3) Sides of the eyes (both sides)

4)   Dark Circles (both sides)

5)   Near the ear

6)   Chin

7)   The tip of the collarbones (both sides)

8)   In the armpits (both sides)

9)   Top of the head in Finnish.

Dr. Hew Len and Dr. Joe Vitale brought this old method to modern audiences' attention, and if you'd like to learn more about it, I suggest reading the following two books: Dr. Joe Vitale is the author of both "Zero limit" and "At zero limit." They are included under the suggested books in the supplementary materials section.

Anyhow, this approach assumes that you are to blame for all problems in your environment since you caused them. Therefore, if you encounter a challenge in your life or learn about a challenge that someone else is facing that troubles you, simply feel the emotion that arises and utter the four phrases. Till you feel at ease once more, repeat them aloud or in your brain.

The four are as follows: I'm sorry

I'm sorry, I do love you.

Many thanks

It is cleared once the bad feeling has left. On everything, you can be certain. The four phrases should be used whenever we feel judgmental, worried, or any other unpleasant emotion because we don't know what is in our subconscious minds. Now try it: I'm sorry, please pardon me, and I love you. Do you feel it? Thanks. It is efficient and effective.

Do I accept that?

- Approach

As long as you don't see it and as long as you think you believe it, a limiting thought can control you. The majority of our limiting ideas reside in our subconscious and exert their influence over us without our conscious awareness. Then, breaking things down and bringing them into our consciousness is incredibly beneficial. You can take the following actions to apply this strategy to eliminate your limiting beliefs:

1. Decide on your limiting thought, such as "I am not deserving of that car"!
2. Money is the source of all evil, and I'm unable to talk in front of others.
3. Reflect on whether you truly believe that concept. If you replied "No," Once the limiting notion has been destroyed, you are finished. Your limiting belief loses influence over you if you refuse to believe it.
4. If you replied "Yes!" Then, consider "why" you hold this belief.

5. Perhaps you will say, "Because I am a bad guy." Then, ask yourself once more, "Do I think I'm a bad person?" Once more if the response is no! You're done now.

6. If you chose "Yes," continue by explaining "why I think I'm a bad person." Finally, you have dismantled the restricting beliefs.

The first step was to eliminate limiting beliefs. Let's go on to the second key now.

Consider Your Intention

When we are clear about what we want out of life, we can make it happen. A better relationship with your children, the love of your life, a new home, a new career, a car, etc. The intention is then set. How do we go about doing that?

You get a piece of paper and jot down your desires. In as much detail as possible. You merely need to record it in writing. Write down every single detail you can think of, such as the brand, model, color, how it feels to sit inside, how it smells, etc., if you want to materialize an automobile.

Then go somewhere peaceful and meditate there. Now, imagine getting what you want. Allow yourself to imagine yourself driving and sitting in your car.

Don't merely replay the visual in your head, here's the trick. You must experience it. Feel how it feels to have what you want, to be driving the car of your dreams, to have others stare back at you as you drive past them. How does it feel in your body?

How does the car feel to the touch? The key is to act as though it has already happened and feel as though you already possess it. You may even replay it in your head as something that took place a year or a week ago. The trick is to make the brain believe that you already own the car and that this has already come to pass.

Spend five to ten minutes contemplating this image. Finally, we must LET IT GO as the final step in setting intentions. Just let it go to the universe, and let it respond to your desire. You don't have to be in control of the outcome, force it, or know how it will manifest in your life. The third step, inspired action, is attained as a result.

Act with Inspiration

You must take inspired action to bring your desire to fruition; you cannot simply sit back and wait for it to fall into your lap. You must respond when the universe calls to you in response to your intention. To take inspired action, think of it as requesting the universe, which will then give you instructions on what to do and when to do it to fulfill your desired intention. By taking inspired action, we are heeding the universe's call. It may serve as inspiration to take action, get in touch with someone, read a book, or tune into a podcast. You may also just feel the need to act when this happens. It's crucial to keep an open mind and to watch out for warning signs. Make sure to investigate anything to which you feel drawn; it might be the universe asking you to do so.

If you take inspired action, you'll get closer than you believe to realizing your desired intention.

The secret codes to manifestation are those. Make use of them now! And your ideal life is just around the bend.

Ways to Increase Vibration

She didn't dance because she was joyful, someone once told me; she did it to make herself happy. Amazingly, that idea is so simple. It follows from a similar assertion on the outward manifestation of interior grace.

These two aphorisms lucidly explain how to alter your vibrational state. For instance, if you are depressed, you will draw unfavorable circumstances into your life. You have the choice to actively alter your frequency by doing an exterior action to avoid it. In the instance of my friend, she decided to dance.

Although it can be, the law of attraction is more than merely bringing luck and wealth. However, it would be a waste to use something so potent only to acquire things that have little cosmic significance. With the law of attraction, you are capable of so much more than that.

To advance to the state of attraction, you must invoke a sense of calm, which you can do by juggling physical exercise with meditation. You can promote that goal by doing a variety of external acts that alter your internal vibration on the inside. This improves your performance coupled with exercise, meditation, and mindfulness. However, there's more. The cosmos has an abundance of resources, thus there are no restrictions on what you can ask for or accomplish.

Rituals

Ritual performance is a further outer manifestation that can be added to an inner grace to fine-tune your vibratory condition.

Rituals are intimately related to the law of attraction in the sense that you instantly resonate at the frequency that attracts exactly what you want when you believe a particular ritual will bring about an event.

Rituals are not antiquated nonsense with no relevance in modern culture. Science has created tools to investigate and test the impact of rituals, and it has produced statistically significant proof that rituals have an impact.

Don't consider rituals to be a feature of prehistoric religions. There are rituals in every religion, including those that are contemporary. Consider moving past these religious pillars. Instead, focus on the coincidence of success following the ritual performance.

Let's use Alexander the Great as an example. He fought the much stronger Persian forces and the lesser provincial armies as he made his way to the center of his enemy's empire, yet he hardly ever lost a battle. Each narrative of his battle is more incredible than the one before it, but they all show how he was able to beat overwhelming odds.

His use of rituals to prepare for each campaign is well known throughout history.

Genghis Khan followed suit. Every major league player, including Joe DiMaggio, Wade Boggs, and others, had their pregame ritual.

The tuning fork of nature is ritual. Together with being attracted, they aid in amplifying the frequency necessary for efficient attraction.

But don't go overboard with the ceremonies. Some people develop an obsession with it, and being in an obsessional state changes the vibration and lessens any possible attractive benefits.

Having a daily morning ritual is an excellent approach to keep yourself in a state of attraction where you are continuously vibrating at the proper vibrational frequency. This regimen should include breathing exercises, meditation, and a little ritual to set the mood.

It takes time and effort to perfect your state of attraction. Both of which require careful cultivation and growth. It is ideal to teach youngsters this vibration so that it becomes second nature to them. Children also find it simpler since they have less mental clutter to sort through. Adults' efforts in life will be greatly impacted by fine-tuning the condition of attraction to the point where it is always in the state of attraction.

Scripting

Actors sometimes have to memorize a series of scripts prepared by scriptwriters when acting in a movie, therefore it seems sensible that when the word "scripting" is uttered, actors, drama, or plays would be the first things that come to mind.

There is nothing special about scripting this time; you are both the writer and the actor.

Writing out your life's tale exactly how you want it to end or writing about a specific event you want to happen to you exactly the way you want it are both examples of the simple approach known as scriptwriting.

Writing out what you're attempting to materialize as though it has already happened.

Writing a script is similar to playing make-believe; you are creating a narrative about your life but writing as if you are already benefiting from what you desire and experiencing the vibration of having it.

You create this complex picture and write this extensive story about how you want something — it might be your life, your day, your relationship, your job, your coffee — the possibilities are endless.

Writing your objectives is quite similar to this, with the exception that this time you're using your imagination to create a creative story.

Using Creativity to Increase Your Success

Using a process called creative visualization, you may bring your aspirations and goals to life. Your life and your prospects of success can be significantly improved if you employ creative visualization techniques correctly. Consider it a form of superpower that you can employ to influence your surroundings, possibly your situations, and bring about desired outcomes. You may utilize it to draw in everything you want in your life, including people, love, work, and money.

Imagine in your mind an action you want to take or an item you want, and you'll draw both of those things to you. While it may appear to some individuals that creative visualization is magic, it is more like daydreaming. The only things at play are the natural rules of mentality and the power of thought.

Unaware that they have this power and are employing it, some people use this in their daily lives. Whether they are aware of it or not, anybody who is successful can attribute their success to their ability to creatively picture what they desire and how their goals have already been achieved.

What functions does it have and why?

That is a fascinating query. Your subconscious notices when you repeat thoughts or think about something repeatedly and begins to accept these thoughts as fact. When that occurs, your actions and habits change along with your thoughts.

Making those adjustments will expose you to new acquaintances, circumstances, and locations, shaping your life and drawing to you exactly what you are imagining.

Thoughts can pass from one person to another. If your ideas are powerful enough, they might inadvertently be picked up by someone who might be able to assist you in achieving your objectives. As you can see, thought is a type of energy that is infused with emotion. Your ideas can alter the equilibrium of the energy around you because of the energy they contain.

How frequently do you find yourself thinking the same thing repeatedly? I would assume that most people do quite a bit. Whether you realize it or not, your mind is always focused on the circumstance you are in and the surroundings. As a result, you can again create the same environment.

When you watch a movie, you may feel as though you've seen it all. Rewatch it now, but this time, alter your perception of the movie. You'll discover that you'll watch the movie very differently and that you'll notice a lot of stuff that you missed the first time. An alternate reality is something you can create.

Once more, this is merely pure natural power that each of us possesses; it is neither magic nor supernatural ability. It's simply that not everyone is aware that they have these abilities, and some people may not use them properly.

Getting Past Strict Thinking

Although creative imagination can greatly improve your life, it's important to keep in mind that no two people are exactly alike. You must be aware that, despite your immense power, it is somewhat constrained. These limitations are internal to us, but they do not possess that power because we cannot all immediately change the same aspects of our lives.

Most of us occasionally impose limits on ourselves and are unable to see beyond a particular area; these limits are a result of our thoughts and beliefs. In other words, we are limiting ourselves to what we already know rather than to what we might learn.

The secret to imaginative visualization is to envision much bigger than we ever ventured to. If you can get over the constraints in your mind, opportunities will increase as you dream broader. Expect no quick fixes; nothing happens overnight. At first, you might just notice a few changes, but the more open your mind and the bigger your thinking, the more will come your way.

You should keep in mind the phrases "patience" and "faith."

Living a Life of Abundance

Using the Law of Attraction, you can draw money into your life. However, much as when looking for love, your thoughts and vibrations must be positive if you want to attract money into your life. By actively taking a more proactive approach to managing your funds, you may set the stage for removing your negative money ideas.

Consider money to be your friend, and see yourself having all the money you require. Imagine holding that cash in your hands and experiencing unlimited financial resources. You can take action to get closer to that state in the interim.

Making plans to pay your payments on time is the most crucial thing you can do to stop worrying about debt. This causes unfavorable vibrations because when people have obligations they can't fulfill—whether they're financial, professional, or personal—they start to feel afraid. Additionally, if you owe money, it is impossible for you to fully concentrate on earning money. Here, the negative negates the positive.

List all of your expenses in addition to this so you may find places where you can cut costs and develop a practical, viable budget.

If all of this seems like a lot of work, consider it removing the detrimental parts of money from your life. By taking the initiative to pay off debt and use your money properly, you are paving the way for abundance. Remember to express gratitude for what you do have rather than wishing for what you lack because both are negative ideas that will lead to similar outcomes.

You're now prepared to apply the Law of Attraction to bring prosperity and abundance to your family and yourself.

The first thing to understand is that wealth is not solely a function of financial resources; you can be affluent in life even if you do not have a lot of money. Being grateful in this situation is important. You will reject money and draw more desperation if you need it—for instance, if you think that winning the lottery will cure all of your financial issues. All those unfavorable ideas are coming to mind once more.

You should keep in mind that you receive exactly what you request. Therefore, you won't acquire the items you might wish to buy with a million dollars if you ask to become a millionaire without also asking for them.

You will receive what you ask for, so be specific in your desires. Here are some suggestions to assist you to maximize your ability to attract money.

Change the way you think about bills and debts

When the bills come in, it's only natural to whine, and those are negative reactions. It is useless to ask "How did we rack up such a hefty amount on the credit card?" You might express thankfulness by telling yourself that you're glad you used the credit card to buy a new washing machine so you can easily keep the family's clothes clean. It may seem strange to express gratitude for a credit card statement, but if you want to apply the Law of Attraction to attract money, you'll need to program your subconscious mind in that way.

Consider the things you have accomplished thanks to the use of electricity, for instance. You've prepared meals for your family, watched television to pass the time, and had light during the night so you could read, use the computer, or check in with pals on Facebook. If you think about it that way, having an electric bill to pay almost feels like a privilege.

Realize How Much Abundance You Have in Your Life Already

Okay, so you might not be a millionaire just yet, but you are wealthy nonetheless. You have plenty of people who are concerned for you, a home over your head, and food to eat.

Simply adopt the attitude that you have a lot to be thankful for and that your life is full of wonderful, practical, and beautiful things, and you will start to attract more plenty because, as you are aware, like attracts like.

You will draw the kind of abundance you desire and have prayed for, whether that is money, things, or perhaps both. If you view yourself as wealthy in non-financial ways, you will inevitably become wealthy in terms of resources. Reprogramming your subconscious is the key to preparing your mind to accept prosperity and abundance. Bad ideas will draw more negative thoughts to you. Therefore, don't assume you lack anything or that, but for fate, you might have become a billionaire. You must consider yourself fortunate to have everything you now possess. If you consider what you now possess to be a lot, then wealth and money will continue to enter your life.

Love cash

It is untrue to suggest that money is the source of all evil. Money is a thing, not a person, and lacks personality traits and a conscience, hence it is not inherently evil. Money itself is not evil; rather, it is how some people utilize it. There is therefore no reason not to appreciate money because it can accomplish a lot of good, and if you have money, you can accomplish a lot of good with it for your family, loved ones, and yourself.

Spend money with pleasure and delight in the products and services you may purchase with it. Develop a relationship with money and learn to appreciate the feel and smell of it. Love the life-improving effects it can have. You must develop a love for it.

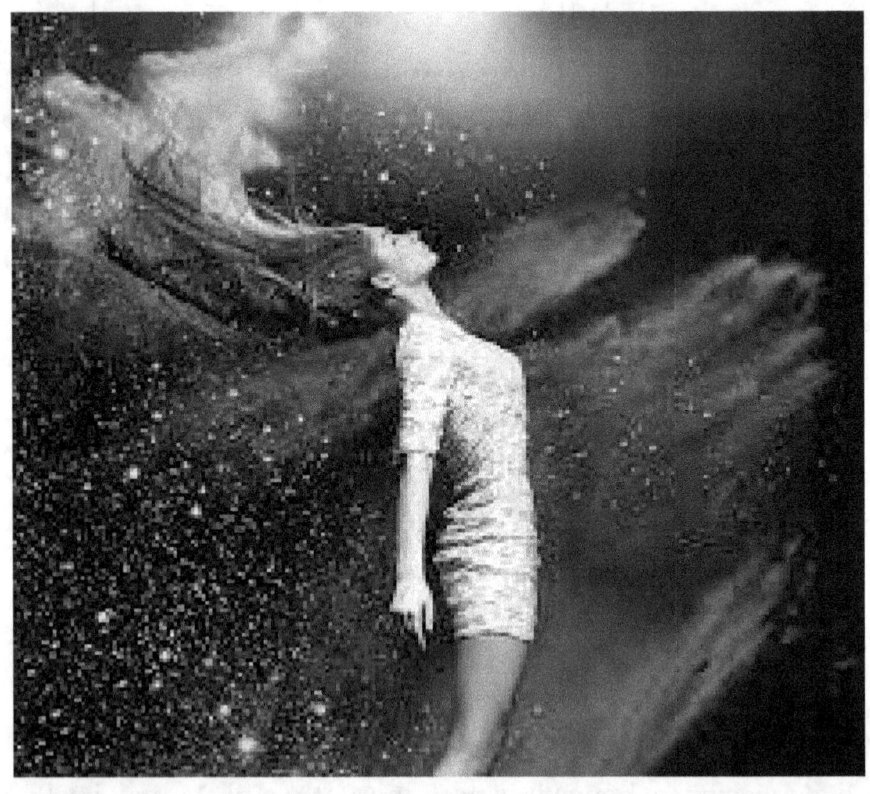

You must think positively about money to send out positive vibes and draw that which you are thinking about into your life. Celebrate its existence and let rid of your negative beliefs about money, bills, and debt. On the other hand, avoid becoming miserly or greedy. These are unfavorable feelings that will keep the money you want at bay.

Above all, avoid feeling envious of others' success. This is a pointless emotion that will not bring you success. It won't help you to succeed if you judge them or feel jealous of their accomplishment. Envy prevents people from obtaining abundance.

The Top 15 Manifestation Secrets

You must first calm your thoughts and unite your mind, body, will, heart, and soul to bring your aspirations and dreams into reality. You might delay or not experience the expected outcomes if your entire being is not consciously aligned with your desire. You might encounter opposition and ultimately unfavorable outcomes. Focus, then!

Your main secret to success is that. You have the power to create everything you want, including wealth, a fulfilling relationship, your ideal home, health recovery, and more. The most important thing is to have faith in your ability to achieve your goals. The greatest discovery of my generation, according to William James, is that a person may change his life by changing his attitudes.

You must maintain your composure and ease as you strive toward your end goal using a combination of your physical, emotional, and spiritual strength. Your desire will materialize into reality!

• Avoid saying "I can't" ever. According to Murphy's Law, "Anything that may go wrong, will go wrong." Instead of letting Murphy's Law control your life, use your judgment.

Never forget the saying "there is a way where there is a will" Therefore, there is always a method to get what you want.

Relax your mind, become lost in your fantasy, and make it come true. Your good vibes will attract the Law of Attraction and help you realize your true goals and aspirations.

Your desires will be obstructed by negativity, which will disrupt your manifestation energy. So maintain mental peace and pay attention to your goals. If you have the motivation to make it happen, nothing is impossible. Even the universe wants to assist you, so you are not alone.

• Holding your head high, stand tall. You should be ecstatic about who you are. You must preserve equilibrium within and a solid basis. You will radiate even more positive energy when you have a positive mindset and dress with confidence. This can help you draw more happiness and prosperity into your life daily.

The Universe is you! You can instantly establish a connection with the universe by drawing on the abundant energy source within of you. Your ability to manifest things increases when you have faith in your dreams.

Your ability to materialize will be messed up if you let stress govern you. Reduce the number of bad feelings in your life. Take the first steps toward your new life. Dress and behave as though you already are the person you aspire to be. Be proud and tall. Feel the triumph.

Make a list of your character strengths and weaknesses. Work now to improve your favorable attributes and eradicate your negative traits. Witness how you will be filled with a lot of wonderful energy. This can help you quickly realize your dreams while also enhancing your individuality.

• Visualize your reality. Keep in mind that the fundamental idea underlying manifesting is that ideas become things. "All that we are is a product of what we have thought," the Buddha said. You must picture what you desire to make it happen.

Additionally essential to the creative process is visualization. You will attract the Universe to fulfill your desires more quickly the more clearly you see them. Give yourself some alone time so that you may unwind and concentrate on your creative visualization. A strong tool for removing any harmful vibrations is visualization. You can visualize it most easily by letting yourself completely unwind. By taking a hot bath or listening to relaxing music, you can unwind. Try to relax your body, mind, and spirit in whatever way you can.

Take a moment to yourself.

Enjoy the now. The more you give your work your whole attention, the more positive vibes you will produce, which will activate the Law of Attraction and help you bring your aspirations to fruition.

Imagination, in the words of Albert Einstein, "is everything. It serves as a sneak peek into life's upcoming attractions.

❖ Create positive energy at all times and embrace wonderful vibrations - When you begin to think positively, you immediately start to vibrate with positive energy. Positive vibrations can be released through daily activities like chatting, imagining, feeling, smiling, and thinking. Do you realize the vibrations you continuously produce? It depends on your attitudes and behaviors whether they are constructive or destructive. You are emitting unfavorable vibrations if you are always anxious, tense, afraid, nervous, etc.

This may disrupt your energy for manifestation. On the other side, if you are at peace within and are relaxed, you will start to vibrate positively. This might attract your desires to materialize through the Law of Attraction. You must direct your energy toward your dominant thoughts and areas of focus if you want to change your current situation. In this manner, you begin manifesting from a higher level of energy, and your wishes manifest swiftly and easily.

You will emanate strong positive energy and allow whatever you want to flow to you naturally when you are at ease, joyful, and self-assured.

❖ Make a "Must Haves" list. You should be aware that every action you take moves you one step closer to the goal. Therefore, it is crucial to first recognize your actual needs, aspirations, and ambitions. You won't be able to concentrate on them unless you know and believe what you truly want. Negative vibrations may emerge from this, delaying the Universe's answer.

To effectively employ the Law of Attraction, take a moment to unwind and consider what it is that you genuinely desire to bring happiness and wealth into your life. You will be able to communicate with your inner self, which can help you decide what is best for you and your future when you are calm. Be precise. Refine. Once you've determined what you want, concentrate on your objectives and make specific progress toward reaching them with the aid of the Universe's abundant source of energy.

Love yourself first. This will give you the self-assurance you need to pursue all of your goals and maintain your focus until they are realized. You must replenish your energy from the plentiful reservoir that is hidden inside of you. You must engage in deep breathing exercises or meditation to access that eternal energy. Your body and mind will relax as a result. You'll learn more about yourself. You can now communicate with your inner self.

You will discover the immense joy and self-assurance that are already inside of you when you connect with who you truly are. Now concentrate on your objectives and consciously employ the Law of Attraction to bring them to pass. Making your desires come to reality is quite simple. It's time for you to give it a go and seize this once-in-a-lifetime chance.

- ❖ Put forth your best effort
- ❖ If you want wonderful things to come your way,

You need to start by giving your all. You must first give your best to receive the best in life. Success cannot be attained quickly.

You have to put in a lot of effort to achieve your goals, whether they be discovering true love or landing your dream career. Before setting any real measures toward accomplishing your goals, you must first calm both your body and mind. You can't relax until your goals are met. Do not lose heart! Today, sow the seeds of your desires. The laws of the Universe will work together to assist you in reaching your goal without fail if you remain committed and put forth the necessary effort. Every time, the initial step must be taken.

Free your thoughts - Before you can materialize, you must first free your thoughts. To assist organize the chaos in your thoughts, you can meditate or engage in deep breathing exercises. Expel all ill feelings. Let it effortlessly float away. When the canvas is empty, you may begin creating your reality. Fill the cup with uplifting ideas.

Keep in mind that if your thoughts are fuzzy, so will the outcomes. Be specific about your desires and aspirations. Never be scared to ask for what you want specifically. Try to imagine how you will feel after achieving your objectives. Will they bring you joy? If not, take another mental break. What would you like? The Universe will assist you in making the proper choices if you can connect with your inner self. Keep thinking until you are certain of your desires, barring any emotional attachment. Meditation is the most effective method for introspection.

The Universe can respond to your inquiries in a state of tranquillity, so connecting to your actual self is simpler than you might imagine. You will also discover the majority of your concerns have answers deep inside. When you are relaxed, you can easily understand the vibrations. Any other method won't work for you. The ability to unwind is a real asset for understanding and self-analysis. To find solutions to your difficulties, try meditation. Take a break from work to relax when you're anxious. When you return to the same issue after a period of silence, you'll miraculously discover the solution you've been looking for.

Achieve your goals every day

"You create your reality as you go along," stated Winston Churchill. Every day, make time for yourself. You can do it whenever and anywhere you please. Just unwind. Focus on your objectives while taking four deep breaths.

You manifest all the time if you are continually thinking.

You can also show up by going about your daily business while thinking, feeling, loving, touching, etc. You can radiate good energy by engaging in a variety of activities. You must act as though your dream has already come true and live in it. By doing this, you can use the Law of Attraction to attract the things you want into your life. All you have to do is contemplate, experience, and accept it.

❖ Unwind - Relaxation is a potent manifesting tool. You must first calm your body and mind to properly concentrate and lose yourself in your dreams. To generate powerfully uplifting vibrations, connect with the abundant source of energy that is already present within you. Higher energy levels will help you create your desires more swiftly and effortlessly.

Express your thanks for all of your aspirations coming true as you unwind. You must have faith that your desires are already coming true. You already possess it if you already think you do. Your wishes will come true because of the cooperation of the universe.

Watch the magic of your dreams quickly become a reality while you sit back and unwind.

• Think positively - According to Charles Haanel, "Like attracts like and the law of attraction states that the dominating idea or mental attitude is the magnet. As a result, the mental attitude will inevitably draw the circumstances that suit it. You must not have any negative ideas or feelings because what you think and feel becomes your reality. Energize yourself with optimism. You'll probably succeed if you tell yourself that you'll succeed no matter what.

You will draw in more positive energy if you are vibrating positively. Therefore, try to unwind and think optimistically. Things will go well for you. Make a note of your flaws and work to eliminate them as soon as you can.

When that happens, you'll be prepared to use the magic and force of the Law of Attraction to bring prosperity into your new life. Buddha once observed, "Your unprotected ideas can hurt you more than your deadliest enemy." Stop allowing negativity to hurt you. You have countless opportunities to improve your life. Try to change your thinking to be more optimistic, and you'll see miracles happen.

❖ Enjoy every moment of your life to the fullest - Your body's vibrations are causing you to materialize at all times. Whichever is more true, you are the best person to judge. You may get rid of negative vibrations and just have positive vibes if you calm down and relax. You are likely to accomplish your objectives more quickly when you manifest from higher vibratory energy. You must take all the necessary steps to maintain your happiness.

Make a list of your goals and go to work on them immediately! Right now, give in to your desires and allow them to raise your vibrational energy. Treat yourself!

Take a trip with your family or friends. Receive a massage. Visit the gym.

Spend some time laughing! Give yourself some delicious food and chocolate. You have the right to experience joy at all times. When you're content, it's easier to concentrate on your objectives and use the Law of Attraction to bring them into reality. Everyone needs "me-time" to engage in their favorite activities.

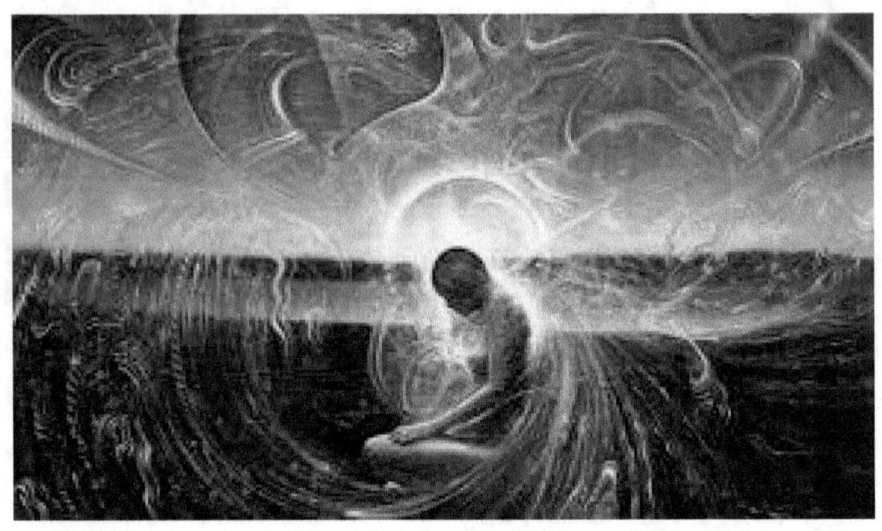

Connect with your spiritual self - You can connect with your inner spiritual self when you are peaceful and relaxed. This will help you become more self-aware. With the aid of your vibrations, you will be able to speak directly with the Universe. You'll be able to find happiness and inner peace as a result. You'll become a happier, more upbeat version of yourself. To comprehend how it feels, you must first mentally experience it. Then, as a reflection of your calm state of mind, you can start to experience manifestations of physical reality, such as riches, success, love, and health.

- ❖ Discover the strength of thanksgiving - The universe is thriving on love, thanksgiving, and kindness. This will speed up the process of drawing in good energy. Thank the universe in the morning for everything you have today. Relax your thoughts and thank the universe for making your wishes come true. Recognize that your desires are currently being fulfilled.

You naturally connect with the universe and the law of attraction when you are overflowing with appreciation. You draw greater prosperity into your life. No matter how minor they may be, be grateful for all the positive things taking place in your life right now. Positive vibrations can be sent out even in silence and picked up by the universe. This is the Law of Attraction's core principle and one of the ways it affects people. Do not beg; instead, only express gratitude if you want to realize your dreams.

Overcome your anxiety, stress, and fear - It's okay to be afraid of the unknown, but try not to let that dread lead to worry and stress. Keep your present from being consumed by bad feelings. Enjoy every minute of your life because it is lovely. Our actions, feelings, and thoughts are all under our control. You must believe in the Universe. Relax your body and mind, and give yourself over to the Universe's countless sources of energy. Scared thinking will cause you to vibrate negatively. This can have a bad effect on your life.

Your manifestation energy will be messed up. Keep your negative feelings, such as uncertainty, fear, desperate worry, depression, etc., at bay. Your negative vibrations will cause you to make unsuccessful or ineffective efforts. Avoid letting your negative ideas rule you, especially if you desperately want something. Instead, fully embrace your dreams and make them a reality. When you begin to think positively, you will draw the Law of Attraction and create your ideal world.

So why are you still waiting? Begin manifesting right now. Just unwind, be precise, and maintain your focus. Exude a positive attitude and visualize everything going your way. Observe how this positive attitude draws you closer to your goals every day. Think in terms of energy, frequency, and vibration to discover the secrets of the cosmos, as stated by Nikola Tesla.

Genuine Freedom and Lasting Contentment

Relying solely on faith either puts a stop to our consciousness' progress or, in response to our spiritual will, invites the soul to step forward as the new source of deeper truth and identity. Consequently, opening up a whole degree of living that was before unimaginable.

Although the highest themes of physical reality are reason and understanding, accepting a spiritual world eventually means giving up access to true freedom and permanent happiness. The logical mind is constrained and unable to experience the delight of believing in a Divinity greater than itself in the absence of a spiritual context for reality.

As a result, it will forever be plagued with a fear of dying and a dread of what lies beyond the grave. Before the advent of a Spiritual Reality, all themes of consciousness may be characterized as viewing the source of consciousness (existence) as the body and mind, but themes after this point perceive the source of consciousness (existence) as the body and mind. The human body and mind are merely outward manifestations of consciousness, which is beyond time and space and represents who we truly are, our actual Self.

More so than something outside of us, the perceived cosmos is something we project upon it. Our perception of the outside world is limited to our consciousness and is related to that theme. Each of us perceives the layers or dimensions of reality differently. Even the concepts of "inner" and "outer," "this" and "that," or subject and object start to converge and finally are discovered to be the same from a larger, non-dualistic perspective. Such a realization transcends logic and enters the mystical and nonlinear worlds.

The mind is compelled to accept the fact that faith and belief determine how we perceive reality, despite its efforts to fight the unfathomable power of believing. The most striking example of this strength of believing is the placebo effect, which defies logic and understanding. The placebo effect is the idea that giving a patient something that does not have therapeutic benefit, but which the patient believes will physically have a healing impact. This is just one of the countless instances of the miraculous that show that faith and belief triumph over knowledge and reason in ways that neither can explain.

At this amazing turning moment, consciousness—our spiritual essence/soul—becomes recognized as our identity, and we let go of our ties to the outside world. When we become aware of our spiritual essence, we have beautiful, limitless access to love and tranquility that are not restricted by our environment. The spirit lives in the regions of true freedom and enduring enjoyment since it is everlasting and therefore survival is already ensured, whereas the human ego lives in perpetual fear and want because of the fear of physical survival.

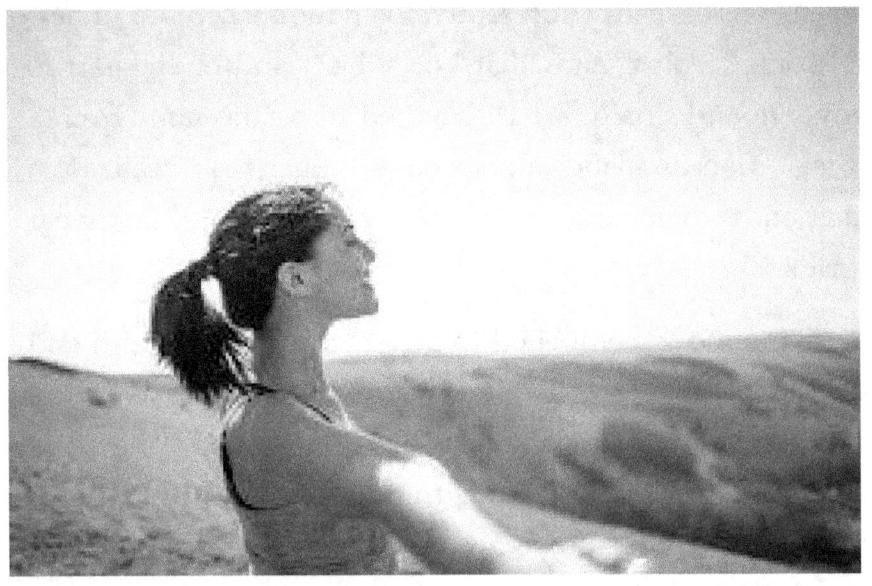

Inner Peace & Love Archetype: Triggers for the Spiritual Seeker: Conditional affection

Root Program: Love and peace come from me.

Love without conditions is transcendence.

The chance to draw love and serenity from the inexhaustible spring within opens up with the dawn of spiritual awakening.

The natural result of ultimately realizing the reality of our spiritual being and discovering thankfulness beyond circumstances is the sensation of inner calm. It would only make sense to choose to view our existence from a perspective that invokes happiness, gratitude, love, and fulfillment if all subjective feelings are a result of an inner choice of perspective. And as we connect with the highest expression of our loving nature, it only serves our interests and those of others, continuing indefinitely.

It is important to keep in mind that what the world refers to as love frequently refers to infatuation, possessiveness, pride, or wishful attachment.

True love is a way to live that is embodied. We start to notice the goodness and love that were previously invisible to us when we enter the frequency of love. True love simply loves because it is in its nature to do so; it does not require a motive to do so.

We begin to finally experience reality at its highest potential when we are in the frequency of love and inner tranquility. If we get beyond the limitations of linear thinking, everything can be seen with love. In many ways, we are experiencing the world as though for the first time.

Colors seem more vivid, we observe damp leaves gleaming in the sunlight as though revealing a magnificent masterpiece, and bumblebees cease to be a bother and instead transform into messengers bestowing their benediction on us. We detect repeated numerals as having significance, and license plates that jump out to us act as signs. No longer is anything merely commonplace or ordinary. The flowers are blooming solely to show us how lovely they are, and the trees are currently twirling for us.

Everything seems to be operating in perfect synchronicity.

Through the freshly discovered lens of love, life is eternally changed into heaven on earth and the magic of Divine Love is visible everywhere we turn. Ironically, it was us who changed; not the world.

Everything has a significance and a purpose in the frequency of love, and everything, even our present circumstances, is giving us advice. Every difficulty or circumstance in life becomes a chance for deeper spiritual enlightenment. Every perceived setback is transformed by Divinity into a redirection.

Accidents and coincidences are no longer occurring. Everything becomes a component of the cosmic conversation between the Creator and humanity. Because of love, everything is seen as being in a loving universe. We readily give into hope and faith even when the significance or purpose of an occurrence in our lives is still unclear because we know it will be revealed to us in due course.

Consciousness perceives love everywhere it turns because it is vibrating at the frequency of love. Even debt is not an enemy of love, as was previously mentioned. Love says to God, "Thank you for allowing me to advance and for giving me a way to repay this tenfold.

My future must be quite promising! If there is perceived rivalry at work or conflict in the world, the thought goes, "Thank you God for giving me the chance to submit, forgive, and put my faith in goodness to use. Everything is in order. What is to be is to be. If this chance wasn't intended for me, it merely indicates that something even better is on the horizon.

From the viewpoint of love, we see that every living thing is an embodiment of a certain theme of awareness and that whatever manifestations others make simply reflect their current nature and not our own.

Hence the adage, "You will recognize them by their fruits." Everything in life must be founded on an internal narrative if there is to be anything objective or personally offensive about it.

For instance, it is merely a projection of another person's internal reality even when it is motivated by rage, hatred, or slander. All suffering is a product of limiting self-created root programs. Pray for your adversaries because they drag themselves down by their own hands, as all great spiritual teachers taught.

These insights enable us to avoid personalizing the suffering of others, which would only cause us to relapse into our limitations. Instead, we have a tremendous amount of empathy, compassion, and tolerance for humanity's dark side. Love honors each person's path through the dark. Love responds to any deemed enemy by saying, "Thank you for the chance to forgive and discover more about myself. What can I do to relieve your suffering? I see you. I am aware of your suffering. I cherish you. As a result, under this topic, compassion for all life becomes the obvious reaction.

Love can express gratitude for anything. Most of life is a gift, and we have little control over it. We do appear to have some choice on how we view this gift of life, though. In light of this, adopting the attitude that everything is going just as it should and that everything is developing for the greater good is the most compassionate course of action. Nothing is an accident, mistake, or coincidence; everything is perfect as it is.

With our limited human perspective, we may not be able to see the perfect justice, balance, and harmony that exists, but we believe in the perfect results of Creation, which may last a very long time after we pass away. Our overall levels of internal freedom, joy, and inner peace dramatically improve when we believe and have faith in such viewpoints.

Every aspect of love's existence is stunning, uplifting, and founded on unwavering faith. Doubt, anxiety, fear, rage, disappointment, expectations, regret, pride, and greed are all relics of the past since they are no longer appealing as viable possibilities. There is enough love to go around. Giving, not taking, is what love is all about.

There is no longer a concern about shortages in this level of consciousness. And love desires to extend generosity and plenty to everybody who is experiencing this fear in the hope that they will also come to understand the generosity of the universe.

Love transcends the physical world and uses intuition to sense energy and essence. Before entering spiritual reality, we could concentrate on observable elements like words, deeds, tone of voice, body language, facial expressions, and even someone's looks. However, love is largely experiencing the subjective energy or essence of another being as it interacts with them (theme of consciousness). It is the distinction between seeing and gut feeling.

To transition from conditional to unconditional love, we must broaden our definition of love to encompass everything that we ordinarily consider to be "unlovable," "tragic," or "ugly" in the world. This third phase transcends preferences entirely and leads to ultimate freedom and enduring enjoyment. Instead, we investigate awareness' of innocence, which embraces the entirety of reality. Love without conditions recognizes that our preferences are not superior to our lack of preferences. Because they are things, they are all equally magnificent.

Only through letting go of the mind's attachments to dualities can unconditional love be realized. This is as opposed to that. Favorable or unfavorable. Therefore, we don't learn to love the "unlovable"; rather, we just learn to let go of the idea that they are unlovable in the first place. All labels are false and originate from artificial viewpoints. Beyond the labels, everything is beautiful the way it is.

Everything in a single, interconnected cosmos is exactly as it should be, without any room for error or mistake. Any other resistance would be an opposition to the cosmos as it is. The spirit focuses on all the evidence of how loved it is, whereas the limited ego opposes love and concentrates on all how it is unloved.

Technically, both viewpoints will seem "correct" and justified, but each will have a distinct experience and result. If we made this one decision, all of mankind could experience complete delight in our existence in a matter of seconds. Because knowing that everything is perfectly in place and not a single hair is out of place thanks to Divine Love makes life an utter joy. We only need to accept it. Access to Divine Unconditional Love is available to everyone.

The sentiments of finally going home to complete security, joy, love, peace, thanks, and indescribable amazement are those of true liberation and enduring pleasure. Everything that is needed to come to understand the reality of Divine Unconditional Love is regarded as irrelevant and worthwhile. Because if that is what it took to get us to where we are right now, then it was ideal and precisely what our consciousness needed to awaken. We are all on the ideal path to remembering how incredibly loved we are by God.

To exist is to already be loved beyond comprehension. The hero's trip through the relativity of ignorance, however, seems to be something we like. As a result, we discover everything about our not-Self only to come back to what was always there but that we hadn't yet noticed.

Unconditional love compassionately recognizes that while some souls accept it more swiftly and resist the temptations of the ego's denial of Divinity, others must stoop to the depths of humiliation and remorse to demonstrate that they are still endlessly loved. In either case, it is all flawless and merely serves to show what is constantly accessible to everyone.

Divine Love, however, cannot compel itself to appear; it must be encouraged. So, t

his essay is a call to genuine liberation and everlasting joy.

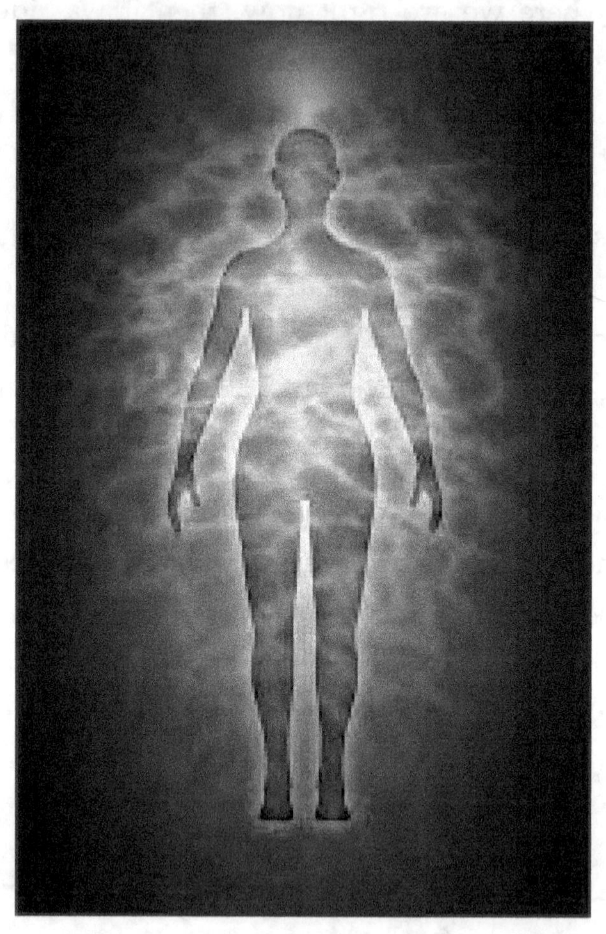

Plan to Raise Your Vibration for 30 Days

Even if you've read through the preceding chapters, you might still feel unsure about how to use this regularly. Setting an intention to do this for 30 days to form a new habit is a fantastic place to start.

You have already read about the daily routine, but before we get into how to choose your affirmations each day, it would be wise to revisit your list of goals to see if any trends could help you organize them into subjects or categories. The majority of people discover that their priorities are either money, work, riches, and relationships, or they are their emotional, mental, and physical health. Other times, you might choose to pursue an education.

Find your categories so that when you create your lists, you can start classifying your demands.

There are a few things you should be aware of before starting the 30-day plan:

This program is intended to be customized to your unique goals and can be used by both novice and experienced affirmation users.

The 30-day plan has a focus for every week.

For those who want to take on a greater challenge, an optional advanced portion is available. Each day is structured around repetitions in the morning, afternoon, and evening. The morning is centered on who you are, the afternoon on what you have, and the evening on what you will do.

Plan for 30 days

Each week is divided into a focus area. Change your emphasis to one that aligns with your aims and objectives. For any of the weeks that don't fit with you, there will be extra emphasis outside of those listed in the plan that you can use to adjust.

Default in the routine

Repeat - Say each of the aforementioned affirmations ten times during each day phase. Take the morning self-focus affirmations, for instance: "I am joyful, I am excellent, and I am eager to start my day."

Repeat each affirmation in that order once; after doing so, there are nine more affirmations left to say. This way of reciting the affirmations is preferred over chanting them repeatedly one at a time. The consecutive chanting of each affirmation enables a pleasant diversity.

Affirmations for the morning are meant to improve your attitude and serve as a reminder of who you are. five affirmations: five when you wake up, five as you're driving to work in the morning.

Afternoon: Concentrate on your possessions and celebrate your achievements. During lunch and each of your commutes, five times each.

Evening: Concentrate on your plans and make sure they come to pass.

five times before bed and five times after dinner

Single or Sequential You can either repeat all of the listed affirmations at once or repeat each one as many times as advised before moving on to the next. As opposed to "I am happy, I am excellent, I am delighted to start my day," for instance, "I am happy, I am happy, I am happy." I'm content, I'm doing well, and I can't wait to get the day going. I'm content, I'm doing well, and I can't wait to get the day going. Although I favor the ladder approach, go with what makes you most comfortable.

You need to incorporate emotions into every affirmation you make. Make it a practice to convey your affirmations emotionally. Usually, when an affirmation is shouted, an emotion is immediately evoked. If not, try an alternative affirmation and observe your reaction.

You are welcome to replace any of the affirmations with ones that are more personal or significant to you. Remember to download your copy of the book's 1000+ affirmations, which are included at the end. To focus this approach on your goals, choose from any of the affirmations included in this book or the free eBook.

Days 1–7: Self-focus

Morning: I'm content, I'm doing well, and I'm eager to get started.

Afternoon: I have a wonderful life, wonderful people in it, and limitless opportunities for happiness.

Evening: I promise to: • Love life and live happily; • Show love frequently, and • Smile every morning.

Day #8–14: Success-Oriented

Morning: I am a wonderful leader; I am successful, and I am driven to succeed.

Afternoon: I have a fantastic career, I have excellent service, and I'm motivated to work hard to succeed.

Evening: I'll be of great value; I'll conquer any obstacles, and I'll accomplish my greatest goal.

Day #15–21:

Morning health focus: I am in good health; I have enough energy; I am perfect, healthy, and entire.

Afternoon: I am in excellent physical and mental health. I am physically robust and powerful. I have a limitless supply of energy.

Evening: I promise to live a long and healthy life, keep my intellect sharp, and carry energy wherever I go.

Day 22 through 30:

Money Focus Morning: I am wealthy; I am committed to wealth, and I am building my net worth

Afternoon: I have access to boundless financial resources, limitless potential for accumulating a fortune, and unobstructed views of lucrative business opportunities.

Evening: I'll have a positive attitude toward money, get money quickly and frequently, and accumulate wealth.

Added Objectives

Focus on Relationships

Morning: I am a wonderful spouse; I am adored by everyone I encounter, and I am committed to fostering wholesome relationships.

Afternoon: I have a devoted partner, best friends, and a caring, supportive family.

Evening: I'll always be a caring, supporting person. I'll create strong relationships.

Confidence Focus for the morning: "I am a role model for others because I am self-assured, dependable, and disciplined."

Afternoon: I can voice my mind with confidence and have great faith in my abilities.

Evening: I will move forward courageously, have confidence in my everyday activities, and be in control of my surroundings.

Advanced Techniques

There are a few things you may add to the 30-day plan if you want to make it more difficult:

- ❖ Use emotional visualization to put yourself in the desired situation. Do this both before bed and in the morning.
- ❖ Incorporate motivational sayings into your morning, afternoon, or nighttime routine. Inspirational sayings

are more potent if they are attributed to an individual who inspires or encourages you.

❖ Express your gratitude for what you already have when you wake up each day. A great method to start the day and prepare your mind for success in whatever focus you are on is this.

❖ You may be thankful at any time of the day; it's not only for the morning. • Put it on paper. Note your feelings of gratitude, affirmations, and quotes.

Plan in advance plan

A single-focus strategy is specifically designed to alter the way you think about one aspect of your life. You must maintain your concentration on one subject for the duration of the plan's 30 days. Use a similar pattern with weekly breaks, but use various affirmations for each routine's theme instead of a different focus for each routine.

This is a fantastic way to alter your opinions and views about a certain aspect of your life. I advise adhering to the suggested plan if you are new to affirmations and then switching to a specific strategy later.

Strategies

As you may have observed, specific affirmations are used to target each day phase. You can utilize a variety of affirmations, all geared toward achieving your goals. For the types of affirmations you choose to utilize during your 30 days of affirmations, I do advise consistency.

If your schedule differs significantly from the majority of ours, your strategy should be modified. It doesn't matter what time of day you say the affirmations; all that matters is that you follow a routine and be consistent every day throughout those times.

Conclusion

Your fundamental beliefs shape your image, which shapes your perspective, which shapes the life you lead, and your outer world reflects it to you. Your life is initially created in your subconscious mind. Your body, mind, and the world in which you live are all one. Your physical body and the physical universe around you are the same things. The non-physical subconscious is an extension of both.

The majority of people are missing their piece of the puzzle, which is how they fit into this universe. Most individuals rarely give their genuine desires much thought; instead, they just consider what they need to do to get through the day or make ends meet. placing others before themselves to a fault, ignoring their dreams, feelings, and emotions.

This is partly because, for countless years, the general populace was convinced that God and life are external to them and that they are unworthy of possessing good things or being affluent. We are all born with sin, nevertheless. We were instructed to fear God and ask for forgiveness. This caused us to lose sight of our internal reality because it was unimportant and we were instead preoccupied with the outside world.

Our ancestors were taught these ideas, which caused us to become detached from reality, and it has persisted ever since. These undesirable concepts are profoundly ingrained in everyone's psyche. There doesn't seem to be any deeper connection to the environment around us. You will never know what shape your puzzle piece takes if you never look in the mirror. To perceive yourself isolated from the rest of reality is to overlook who you are on the inside.

You can see who you are when you learn to look inside and understand how the interior connects to the outside world. How do you fit in and the best method for you to achieve a happy, successful, and rewarding life? You already possess all the love and joy you could ever want.

Most people forget about themselves and have a very low opinion of themselves since they tend to look outside of themselves for answers. People don't believe they are deserving enough to realize their dreams. We are shown and indoctrinated at a young age that happiness comes from things outside of ourselves.

Our interior reality is not demonstrated to be more significant or real than the external world. But we try to use things outside of ourselves to satisfy our interior contentment. The idea of cause and effect was demonstrated to us; for instance, if you get this new toy or achieve that objective, you would thereafter feel glad.

Because the outside world is transient and always changing, that kind of bliss never lasts. We are taught to look outside of ourselves, yet we don't realize how distorted our perceptions of reality are. To fulfill your dreams, happiness is a prerequisite.

Your inherent truth is static and independent of the world around you. We can learn to take control of those feelings and produce more lasting happiness by realizing that most of our true life is experienced through our thoughts and feelings.

We now know that polarities in life can be used both ways. Since a cause and an effect are always equal, we can learn to produce a positive mood first to attract more positive things to us. It's internal to life.

Taking the necessary actions to achieve fulfillment or achievement is not enough. It is important to strike a chord with them first, and then go forward from there.

To succeed, you must first feel and believe that you are succeeding. This knowledge must reside in your heart, which is the source of all of your emotions.

You are more real within than the outer world could ever be, and your body, existence, and internal truth of your ideas and feelings are your genuine gifts. Everything you take for granted as real would not exist without you.

Your consciousness creates the reality of your life. Success and contentment come from inside, but they also require abilities that may be developed. We must learn to follow our instincts and to perceive the environment as a reflection of ourselves to understand that we have a hand in shaping the experiences we have.

We must first transform ourselves before we can affect the surrounding environment. We must first learn how to help ourselves before we can help others. Until we learn to cure ourselves, we cannot contribute to the healing of the planet. What we have yet to learn, we cannot impart to others.

Your reality is mirrored back to you from your head and emotions. To alter your world, you must first learn to accept what is, and then you must adopt a new way of thinking to inspire a shift in your feelings and the formation of new beliefs. Your perspective will alter if you develop new habits and a new mindset.

It can require persistence and time. Your friends are repetition and practice; they aid in the creation of a new universe. a universe that you create by first having faith in it. Once you observe the manifestation as a result of your belief, your belief will be strengthened.

You already do this, but you haven't watched yourself close enough to notice it yet, and you don't do it on purpose.

Your ability to live more fully and purposefully depends on your ability to see yourself and how your mind functions. The average person typically has a negative outlook on life, and it is human nature to get lost in our thoughts and imagination. The only moments we are not engrossed in our imaginations are when we are concentrating on a task, solving issues, or taking pleasure in a physical activity like watching a fantastic movie or playing a game.

Otherwise, we all live in our imaginations during the gaps between activities like driving a car or performing other menial tasks. Our natural tendency is to fret about the past, worry about the future, and pass judgment on people or circumstances. By accelerating and having to prevail in mental debates, among other things, we recreate or make new circumstances.

We can far more readily comprehend the control our brains have over us when we can watch ourselves getting naturally carried away by them. The power of the imagination should not be taken lightly. We can decide whether or not to think better thoughts.

must decide to see the dreams and goals we want, imagine them, and experience their emotional manifestation.

Learn to be aware of how often you use your imagination and to pay attention to how strong your anger feels when it is directed at someone or an uncontrollable circumstance. It seems very genuine.

By realizing that you already utilize your imagination continuously, you can learn to make conscious decisions to think of better things. Learn to replace your negative ideas with your goals, keep them in mind frequently, and rewire your thoughts to be positive. As much as you can, try to live in a happy, goal-oriented imagination. By intentionally employing it, you may banish the majority of unfavorable thoughts and brighten your days. Making the imagination work for us rather than against us is the aim.

Your business's success is dependent on the vision you have for it and the actions you take to make that vision a reality. Therefore, consider what "the ultimate" outcome of running a successful firm is and how that should affect how you act and think. Regarding all I have discovered and my progress to date. I've reached the following conclusion, and I make an effort to live up to it.

The customers you serve are more important to a successful business than anything else. They are the root of the problem and the reason the company exists. Therefore, success entails looking out for the interests of the client, whether or not the solution is advantageous for you. You must point them in the direction of where they can discover a solution if you are unable to assist them in doing so.

You must learn to be sincere, recognize when to take a step back, and understand that this person needs your assistance whether they need it or not. They'll respect you just as much as if you provided them with your services, and they'll recommend you to others. Whatever industry you work in, if it involves money, it involves people.

Because of this, no matter what kind of business you are in, you must always operate in a service-oriented manner if you want to expand. You can serve more customers and become more profitable the more people-oriented you become. The side effect is money.

The vision is what matters, not the amount of money. It is about the path you take to reach your goals.

Being original is necessary if you want to thrive, assist others, and have work that is both financially rewarding and personally meaningful. being authentic, bringing your personality to work, and bringing your passions to work. You'll be more motivated to expand your business and do more of what you love if you can be authentic in your profession. People will seek you out expressly because they can sense your confidence and passion if you can love what you do.

Consider how you would behave and think if the circumstance you were trying to create were already real. You must portray the role. You should make an effort to spend as much time as you can in that world, realistically speaking. Successful thinking, feeling, and speaking.

Things don't just happen for no cause; you must first resonate with them to create them. To think from the end is to live in the end.

Success must be a way of life for you. You must orient your thoughts in the direction of goal fulfillment. You can think creatively, while most people spend their days worrying about various issues without ever deciding to direct their attention in a constructively forward-looking manner.

Your feelings are influenced by your thoughts, and unrelated worries might cause a stress frenzy. Learn to shift your attention from worrying to achieving your goals. Your subconscious will begin to shift as you regain control of your focus, and then your behaviors will follow. Your path to success will start to take shape in front of you as your actions adapt to match your desires.

True faith entails setting goals for your internal reality and taking the necessary efforts to achieve them. The environment around you will change as you believe it and move on.

To keep your attention on the desired result, utilize affirmations frequently and daily meditation.

You must devote everyday thought to achieving your goals, just as you must do for breathing, eating, and sleeping. To learn more and grow as a person, you must regularly take action. As you advance, so will your company. Walk in the direction of the target.

The change you wish to see in the world must start with you. Your heart and mind are at the core of who you are. With the appropriate focus, your life and the success of your business will advance, just like the sun and planets do as they travel through space. The secret is to learn how to direct your attention ahead, and the way to accomplish so is by practicing and repeatedly reminding yourself how life functions.

The ability to enter your subconscious, examine who you are, how you think, what you want from life, and how figure out how to get there make meditation one of the most beneficial activities you will ever undertake. It is the most popular activity successful individuals around the world perform, especially when combined with meditation's calming effects.

The value of repetition and deliberately setting aside time to concentrate on your goals cannot be overstated. You need to understand your mind since it has tremendous control over your life and you need to use it to your advantage.

to assist in leading you forward in time and space to the location on which you are focusing. You are the Law of Attraction, quantum physics, the atom, and the electron, your ambitions, and anything you focus on and feel the strongest about.

Until your perspective matches the world around you, choose to see things from that perspective. You must be adamant, possess a mind over matter, and have faith in your abilities and aspirations. If a situation is stressful, select a different way to look at it, add a fresh viewpoint, or choose not to think about it at all.

When you genuinely alter your viewpoint and thinking, the world will reflect this change in you, but only after your subconscious mind has given the adjustment its approval.

According to what I've heard, an airline pilot must control the plane 95% of the time and only 5% of the time. To attain our goals, just as in life, we must constantly refocus on them. This is similar to meditation practices in that we must continuously refocus our thoughts and breathing to enter a deep state of meditation.

You must treat your company as if it were your kid because you are one with it. Consider it positively, be grateful for it often, and picture it as a child. Plan the right course of action to promote its expansion. Set objectives and deadlines for achieving them.

Pay attention to your thoughts and the way you talk to other people about who you are and what you do.

Make every effort to control the thoughts and words you use since you are projecting your internal reality. By doing so, a new cause and effect will be produced. Your surroundings reflect your subconscious, therefore as you concentrate on developing, your reality will eventually show you the results of your efforts. Being the visionary of your life can help you to develop patience, love yourself more, love thinking, appreciate the journey, and recognize the power of your intellect.